What You Really Want to Know
About Life with Dementia

by the same authors

Evidence-Based Practice in Dementia for Nurses and Nursing Students
Edited by Karen Harrison Dening
Foreword by Alistair Burns
ISBN 978 1 78592 429 3
eISBN 978 1 78450 797 8

Dementia, Culture and Ethnicity
Issues for All
Edited by Julia Botsford and Karen Harrison Dening
Foreword by Alistair Burns
ISBN 978 1 84905 486 7
eISBN 978 0 85700 881 7

Young Onset Dementia
A Guide to Recognition, Diagnosis, and Supporting
Individuals with Dementia and Their Families
Hilda Hayo, Alison Ward and Jacqueline Parkes
Foreword by Wendy Mitchell
ISBN 978 1 78592 117 9
eISBN 978 1 78450 383 3

of related interest

A Pocket Guide to Understanding Alzheimer's Disease
and Other Dementias, Second Edition
Dr James Warner and Dr Nori Graham
ISBN 978 1 78592 458 3
eISBN 978 1 78450 835 7

Enhancing Health and Wellbeing in Dementia
A Person-Centred Integrated Care Approach
Dr Shibley Rahman
Forewords by Professor Sube Banerjee and Lisa Rodrigues
Afterword by Lucy Frost
ISBN 978 1 78592 037 0
eISBN 978 1 78450 291 1

Telling Tales About Dementia
Experiences of Caring
Edited by Lucy Whitman
ISBN 978 1 84310 941 9
eISBN 978 0 85700 017 0

Excellent Dementia Care in Hospitals
A Guide to Supporting People with Dementia and Their Carers
Jo James, Beth Cotton, Jules Knight, Rita Freyne, Josh Pettit and Lucy Gilby
Foreword by Tommy Dunne
ISBN 978 1 78592 108 7
eISBN 978 1 78450 372 7

What You Really Want to Know About
Life with Dementia

REAL STORIES AND EXPERT
ADVICE FOR FAMILY, FRIENDS
AND PEOPLE WITH DEMENTIA

**Karen Harrison Dening, Hilda Hayo
and Christine Reddall**

Foreword by Keith Oliver

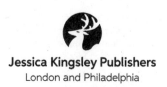

Jessica Kingsley Publishers
London and Philadelphia

First published in Great Britain in 2023 by Jessica Kingsley Publishers
An imprint of Hodder & Stoughton Ltd
An Hachette Company

4

Disclaimer: The information contained in this book is not intended to replace the
services of trained medical professionals or to be a substitute for medical advice.
You are advised to consult a doctor on any matters relating to your health, and in
particular on any matters that may require diagnosis or medical attention.

A CIP catalogue record for this title is available from the British Library and the
Library of Congress

ISBN 978 1 78775 695 3
eISBN 978 1 78775 696 0

Printed and bound by CPI Group (UK) Ltd, Croydon, CR0 4YY

Jessica Kingsley Publishers' policy is to use papers that are natural, renewable and
recyclable products and made from wood grown in sustainable forests. The logging
and manufacturing processes are expected to conform to the environmental
regulations of the country of origin.

Jessica Kingsley Publishers
Carmelite House
50 Victoria Embankment
London EC4Y 0DZ

www.jkp.com

Contents

Meet the Editors

PROFESSOR KAREN HARRISON DENING

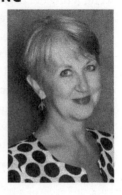

Karen has more than 40 years' experience in nursing, most of those being in dementia care in a variety of settings and contexts. She is Head of Research and Publications at Dementia UK. She gained her PhD at University College London in advance care planning and end-of-life care in dementia. Through her role at Dementia UK, she is a collaborator, co-applicant and expert advisor to several national and international research studies. She served on both of the National Institute for Health and Care Excellence (NICE) dementia guideline committees. Her research interests are dementia care, case management, carer resilience, palliative and end-of-life care, and advance care planning.

DR HILDA HAYO

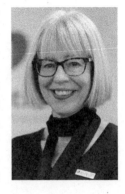

Hilda became Chief Admiral Nurse and CEO for Dementia UK in 2013. A dual-registered nurse, over the last 36 years she has held senior positions in clinical services, hospital management and higher education. Hilda is particularly proud of setting up and leading a nurse-led Younger People with Dementia service in Northamptonshire and still provides specialist advice and support to families. Her doctorate focused on behavioural variant frontotemporal dementia and how this affects families. She has also written a book on young-onset dementia with two colleagues, published in 2018.

CHRISTINE REDDALL

Christine, a qualified nurse since 1973, has worked in many different settings. She became a community Macmillan nurse in 1991, fulfilling an ambition to work in palliative care. Completing her degree in 1997, she specialised in care homes delivering palliative care education to carers. Realising that people with dementia and those with learning disabilities rarely accessed good palliative and end-of-life care, she concentrated her efforts on enabling this. In 2012, Christine's eldest daughter, Anna, 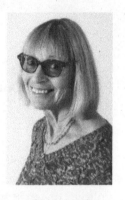 aged 37, was diagnosed with a type of young dementia called behavioural variant frontotemporal dementia (BvFTD). Anna died aged just 42. Since then, Christine has used her experience gained from both her professional and personal perspective to help promote awareness of young dementias.

Contributors to This Book

PEOPLE WITH DEMENTIA AND FAMILY CARERS

- Sylvia Bates
- Surinder Bangar
- Molly Barry (pseudonym)
- Theresa Clarke
- Bridget Culson (pseudonym)
- Rob Garrett
- Jane Hall (pseudonym)
- Alan Hewitt
- Brian Humphreys
- Gina Hyde (pseudonym)
- Alfie Jones (pseudonym)
- Wendy and Sarah Mitchell
- Liz Murphy (pseudonym)
- Christine Reddall
- Marion Small (pseudonym)
- Nula Suchet
- Jack and Caroline Worth (pseudonyms)

SPECIALIST COMMENTARY

- Dr E. Joanna Alexjuk
- Dr Janet Carter
- Jo-Ann Dawson
- Professor Tom Dening
- Dr Rheinhard Guss
- Dr Malsha Gunathilake
- Professor Rowan H. Harwood
- Professor Karen Harrison Dening
- Professor Julian C. Hughes
- Dr Jacqui Hussey
- Professor John Keady

- Professor Jill Manthorpe
- Dr Kirsten Moore
- Dr Manisha Ray
- Dr Malarvizhi Babu Sandilyan
- Dr Graham Stokes
- Professor Elizabeth Sampson

ADMIRAL NURSES

- Zena Aldridge
- Loraine Butterworth
- Fiona Chaabane
- Lucy Chamberlain
- Dr Jacqueline Crowther
- Maggie Fay
- Dr Hilda Hayo
- Deborah Hutchinson
- Stuart Kennedy
- Rachael Lowe
- Kerry Lyons
- Saul Mason
- Angela Moore
- Chris O'Connor
- Tom Rose
- Nikki Rowe
- Rachel Thompson
- Sharron Tolman

Foreword

As a lifelong avid reader, I continue to read a lot, but due to my dementia I remember little of what I read. However, this book is an exception to this as it captured my interest throughout and drew me into the world of others affected by dementia, alongside learning so much from the wisdom and experience of the health and social care professionals and academics.

The authors have cleverly used a structure for the book which I resoundingly applaud, that of starting with the words of those who are affected by dementia, be it with a diagnosis or as a family carer, then taking those words and placing them alongside commentary from eminent academics and professionals. Our understanding is then expanded with very sound and clear guidance from Admiral Nurses. I do hope that this book contributes to the drive to fund and recruit more Admiral Nurses – we *do* need them, and my wife always readily acknowledges the excellent support she receives from her Admiral Nurse.

I also applaud that the book takes the reader from examining the importance of an early, accurate, professionally delivered diagnosis through to the need to compassionately support the person with dementia and those closest to us at the end of life, with a comprehensive insight into life in-between.

I personally relate very closely to so much within the case studies but two particularly resonate at the moment, one being Caroline's description of the rollercoaster and the second Eric's account about apathy especially relating to travel, something my wife and I have always enjoyed and more so since we retired, but which now my dementia is making far more difficult.

In the 11 years since being diagnosed with Alzheimer's I have read many books on dementia and seldom has one taught me as much, moved me as far, or inspired me more than this one to continue to try and do 'my bit' in the realm of activism and awareness raising.

Keith Oliver
Honorary Doctor, Canterbury Christ Church University, Alzheimer's
Society Ambassador & Kent & Medway Dementia Envoy

Preface

As you read this book, it will be hard not to notice and feel the diverse and complex emotions that thread themselves throughout each case study. All these emotions resonate strongly with me as I experienced every single one throughout the five years of watching my daughter, Anna, endure the profound effects of young-onset dementia.

Reading through the case studies, it struck me how often family carers mentioned the feeling of guilt. For me, guilt was ever present, shrouding so many aspects of my caring role. Guilt was the hardest emotion to deal with, and even now, four years after Anna's death, it still has the power to raise its ugly head and remind me of all the times I felt I had failed my daughter.

When I was asked to contribute to editing this book from a carer perspective, I felt privileged that I was able to offer something positive from my experience and help others who are going through the dementia caring role.

What I didn't realise was how much this book was going to help me. I have been amazed at how much I have gained both from reading the very personal case studies and from the explanation and advice offered by the specialist commentator and the Admiral Nurses. Had I had access to a book such as this when I was floundering from the physical and emotional impact of caring for Anna, I am sure it would have helped tremendously.

Christine Reddall

ADMIRAL NURSING

Admiral Nurses are specialist dementia nurses who are continually supported and developed by Dementia UK and provide life-changing support for families affected by all forms of dementia. Admiral Nurses can help families to understand dementia and its effects, and help them to develop the confidence to manage their future with dementia. The nurses have time to listen to the person who contacts them, assess the person's needs and provide the expertise to solve issues that may arise when a family member has dementia. Admiral Nurses specialise in helping families to manage complex issues that can arise as a result of dementia including distress, relationship and role changes, communication difficulties and changed behaviour or personality. In addition to being specialist dementia nurses, some Admiral Nurses also specialise in different areas of dementia including young-onset dementia, Lewy body dementia, frailty, end-of-life care, diverse communities, learning disability, acute care, primary care and long-term care. This book highlights the work of some of our Admiral Nurses in a range of settings and provides an example of their specialist knowledge and skills in a range of situations.

So why are we called Admiral Nurses? The family of Joseph Levy CBE BEM, who founded the charity Dementia UK, named the nurses. Joseph had vascular dementia and was known affectionately as Admiral Joe because of his love of sailing. His family wanted to make a difference for families living with the effects of dementia and set up the charity to support and develop specialist dementia nurses, and they decided to call us Admiral Nurses.

The number of Admiral Nurses across the UK is steadily increasing, and they work in a range of services including the community, GP practices, NHS hospitals, hospices and care homes. There are still areas of the UK that don't have access to a local Admiral Nurse service and for these families we have the Admiral Nurse Dementia Helpline (0800 888 6678 or email on: helpline@dementiauk.org), open seven days a week and staffed entirely by specialist dementia nurses. In addition, we have Admiral Nurse Clinics (Closer to Home[1]) where a virtual appointment can be booked with a specialist dementia nurse.

Dr Hilda Hayo, Chief Admiral Nurse

---

1   www.dementiauk.org/get-support/closer-to-home

Introduction

Welcome to this book that aims to give families affected by dementia an opportunity to voice their questions and concerns. There are many options now for people with dementia and their families to gain answers to their many and varied questions on dementia from the point when they feel 'something is not quite right' to understanding how to get a diagnosis right through to best care at the end of life. At Dementia UK, the 'home' of Admiral Nurses, we provide information, advice and support to families affected by dementia when faced with a myriad of issues, questions and concerns. As well as providing the Admiral Nurse Dementia Helpline (details in the Admiral Nursing section at the beginning of the book), we work with many host organisations to provide Admiral Nurses who work across a wide range of health and social care settings. In developing the concept for this book, we wanted to provide a resource that was similar to the Admiral Nurse Dementia Helpline and place the focus on what the person with dementia and their family carers felt were the most important questions for them: what they wanted to know and not what professionals think they should know, as is the basis for many self-help books in this field.

We wanted families affected by dementia to steer the content of the book. This seemed fine in principle, but that then gave us the task of asking families affected by dementia what questions were most important to them that they felt should feature in the book. Many families state, 'If only I knew this back then...' or 'If only I could go back knowing what I know now...' – would this knowledge have made a difference? They and we will never know, but this seemed like a good approach to enable those families to benefit from their experiences but in a new way.

So, key to developing the book was to ask people with dementia and family carers and supporters: in living with dementia, what do you want to know? We hope this book proves of value to the readers.

(If you wish to know how we went about asking families affected by dementia what they wanted to know, please see the appendix at the end of this book.)

Professor Karen Harrison Dening

Dr Hilda Hayo

Christine Reddall

A NOTE ON TERMS USED

We realise that there will be differing opinions on names and terminology used in this book. We have tried to balance this while also aiming for consistency in some of the terms, such as 'people with dementia' and 'family carers'. It is not our intention to cause offence or diminish the impact of what it is like to be diagnosed with dementia or for a family member or friend close to that person.

CHAPTER 1

'Discovering my mother through Alzheimer's'

LIFE STORY

Surinder Bangar

My parents were admitted into hospital during the first wave of the pandemic; both were confirmed as Covid-19 positive. Three days after their admission, my father passed away. In the initial stages after his death, my mother was unable to remember what had happened and would ask, 'Where is your father?' She knew there was something that she should know, yet she seemed unable to access this information. It felt important to respond in ways that would make sense for her and to talk in Punjabi to help her feel comfortable and to make things easier for her. In our home, we usually refer to my mother as 'Bibi' and I'll sometimes use this term in the text.

Eventually, after months of agonising grief, Bibi would nod when I'd say, 'He had a chest infection.' Talking about my father's illness and death began to provide a way for Bibi to describe what happened when other people close to her passed away. She started to talk about our Baba (grandad) and how he'd passed away unexpectedly: 'We'd just been to see him at the hospital and the next day he was dead.' Then something remarkable began to happen. My mother began to show us how to cope with bereavement and how to appreciate our lives. Drawing on these memories of my grandad, Bibi would start to talk about family, India and coming to England. Bibi would explain that, culturally, she married into and belonged to my father's family; she spoke fondly of Baba and how much he did for her both in India and in England. How much he did for everyone in the family, how hard he worked, how much he used to read to educate himself. Baba was a bricklayer, and she talked about his work in India and about the building projects he worked on in England. It was Baba who was able to get the necessary paperwork to enable my father to come to England to work. Bibi said that our father had been pestering Baba to arrange for her and the three of us in India to join him. She said my father kept saying he was missing his family. I learned that in 1966, when my mother came over to England to join my father, it had been prompted by the age of my oldest sister who was eleven; apparently, there was a restriction which meant that after this age she would not have been able to gain entry as easily. Bibi said she had refused to join without bringing all three children with her. As she immersed herself in describing her past, Bibi's sharpness and humour would permeate these stories.

Bibi's eyes would light up as she described our heritage and when she talked about houses in India that she had lived in. My parents' generation lived through Partition, and Bibi began to talk about the district of Lyallpur where she lived, which subsequently become part of Pakistan. Bibi remembered the date of Partition and described how people all used to live together and work together, and there was a sense of how happy she was as a child. She talked about her own siblings and told me that she was the eldest – I had never known anything at all about her own family. I found out that her family home was extensive and surrounded by land. She said she was around eleven or twelve when Partition happened, and she would go on to describe some of the terrible things she lived through. There was so much sadness deep in her eyes and her voice. As she continued, she would expand upon Partition as arising from problems of government and politicians, and would comment on the state of India now and what would be better.

In talking about her early life, Bibi started to talk about my father. At these points, she would recount stories of their life in India, about his work and how he used to travel on the train to work. She told me the times of the daily trains to/from the village where they lived and about the food that they used to prepare for them. Cows and milk featured heavily and how it was a tradition to drink hot milk in the evenings, with families sitting outdoors and chatting into the evening. The tradition of hot milk continued in my parents' lives as their evening routine consisted of a nightly mug of hot milk. My mother's view remains that the milk is different and better in India.

Relatives recounted how much our parents did for them, how they generously helped to support them when they were younger, both in India and in this country. As she did when describing my Baba, my mother started to talk affectionately about my father and about the many things he did for family members and how he cared for her when she first came to England. Houses formed a recurring part of conversations, and she talked about the house we initially lived in with my Baba and our extended family before my parents bought their own home. Bibi described how my father used to go to the pub after work with his brothers and two friends who were also from India. She would say, 'Your father worked hard in his life, I didn't mind him going out and it is important to enjoy life after working so hard.' Underneath, I felt the echoes of how hard it must have been for both of them to make a new life, in a new country, arriving in the 1960s against a backdrop of increasing immigration controls.

It seemed as though my mother was going through what was most striking to her in their lives together. At other times, she would talk about going out to work as a machinist. My mother worked in a factory for over twenty years making waterproof garments. She went out to work, navigating getting a bus there and back on her own. When she first started, she was the only Asian woman working in the factory. My mother described the friends she made and how they all helped her. The women at work helped her with learning some English.

Discovering my mother's story

I had never heard my mother describe her early life so vividly, and I discovered family history that I had never known before. It felt a privilege to hear her talking and reflecting. In some ways, the conversations were a celebration of their lives, her life and her history and what mattered most to her. Where possible, I started to do voice recordings on my phone when she was underway with a memory – sometimes this worked and sometimes it didn't as it depended on how she felt at any moment. We started to share what Bibi was talking about with our relatives when they rang and they wanted to know more – they would say, 'Your mother knows everything about our families and India; make sure you write this down and let us know because we also don't know some of this.' I started to do short video recordings on my phone because video was better to capture her enthusiasm, her expressions, her workings out and the aliveness that she demonstrated when telling stories. In some of the videos, my mother is doubled up in laughter recounting anecdotes or describing family episodes. It has been a joy to see my mother enjoying herself. I would start by asking her, 'Is it OK to record this so that I can show other members of our family?' My mother had grown up in an extended family setting, with skills and knowledge being passed on through the generations. Being able to introduce this intergenerational aspect connected with Bibi, and I feel it helps Bibi to feel valued, particularly when Alzheimer's continues to take so much away from her.

I replayed a video to Bibi when she was explaining how to make samosas. She laughed and said, 'There, you've got this now; when I'm dead, you will always have me telling you this.' My mother didn't go to school in India, and while she is able to read and write some Punjabi, she doesn't independently write or record her ideas in a formal way. Word of mouth has acted as a strong tradition to learn skills and acquire knowledge. It struck me that these mini recordings provide a tangible record in a way that we didn't have previously. Family members participated in different ways: my sister digitised a collection of photos; my brother-in-law converted an old VHS tape to a CD format so that the footage could be better preserved; my aunt bought some Punjabi books of short stories for my mother to read; DVDs of my mother's favourite movies and television shows, both English and Punjabi, were added to the growing repository at home. I found that it was important to follow cues from my mother. For example, sometimes she would be receptive to photographs and at other times she wanted to switch off from these and found them confusing or upsetting. Things are continuing to evolve. I am continuing to make videos, audio recordings, notes and photos about my mother and her memories and observations. Each time, her stories and anecdotes seem like a gift to be treasured. In looking back, she is also looking at the present and to the future.

I feel acutely aware that my parents' generation is coming to an end. It feels vital to preserve my mother's memories and observations, and to share these as a family. They are acting as a helpful conversation aid with my mother. My father is no longer with my mother to provide a safe anchor to their shared histories. I am working on what we can do to preserve my mother's memories in the face of these being slowly eroded through Alzheimer's. My mother's memories are inextricably connected to my father, and it feels as though I am continuing to discover them both through my mother's eyes. However, we are not just our memories, or even other people's memories of us. There's understanding and wisdom and beliefs and the changes we make in the world around us. In caring for my mother, I am encountering myself and she is continuing to teach me. I am thankful to her for all that she has done for us and continues to do.

SPECIALIST COMMENTARY

John Keady, Professor of Mental Health Nursing and Older People, University of Manchester/Greater Manchester Mental Health NHS Foundation Trust

Life story: why are stories important?
Telling stories and story-making is integral to human consciousness and lived experience. Indeed, telling stories – in whatever language we are most familiar with – is part of what it is to be human and to identify with a shared cultural and linguistic heritage.

Stories perform a valuable social role and function as they connect us through time to our past, our present and our future. We see evidence of this connection in the shared life story in this chapter when, as a person with dementia, Bibi started to talk about her husband. As shared by Surinder, 'At these points, she [Bibi] would recount stories of their life in India, about his [her husband's] work and how he used to travel on the train to work. She told me the times of the daily trains to/from the village where they lived and about the food that they used to prepare for them.' And later, when Bibi and her family located from India to England, the simple but profound insight, that '[t]he women at work helped her [Bibi] with learning some English'. This storied narrative jumps out from the page. Even though we may not hold the same cultural heritage as Bibi and her family, we can identify and empathise with the shared life experiences, possibly transposing them on to our own lives and times when we have felt separated from those closest to us and/or displaced from a community where we once had a sense of belonging. Stories – and life stories in particular – are individual, relational, (auto) biographical, meaningful and universal. They are also highly personal.

Life story: how is it useful in dementia care?

As stories define who we are and how others understand and see us, it is perhaps no surprise that in dementia care, life story has long held an important place and positioning. There are perhaps two main reasons for this. The first is that in Alzheimer's disease, for example, the autobiographical memory of people with dementia will become significantly compromised with the passage of time and the person will find it more and more difficult to remember and share stories about their own life in a chronological order and in a way that is always understandable to others. Stories and experiences from the past can become entangled with experiences and life in the present. Second, without a grasp on who we are, and an ability to clearly articulate this to others, an individual's personhood can become devalued and their actions misunderstood and stigmatised. For people with dementia, therefore, one of the inherent risks is that, without a life story that can be remembered and told solely by/about the person him- or herself, that person's sense of self and personal identity will be significantly compromised. In the 1990s, this threat was acknowledged by Professor Tom Kitwood – who was a highly influential social psychologist in dementia care working (at the time) at the Bradford Dementia Group in the UK – in his important book *Dementia Reconsidered: The Person Comes First* (Kitwood 1997). In that book, Kitwood (1997, p.56) said that 'biographical knowledge about a person [with dementia] becomes essential if that identity is still to be held in place' and he suggested that in order to maintain the identity of a person with dementia, life story work was foundational to undertaking person-centred care. Almost 25 years later, the importance of this statement for care, research and policy practice has not diminished at all.

Life story: why is it important?

For dementia care practitioners, the development and compiling of a life story helps to uphold the personhood and identity of people with dementia. The mechanics of undertaking life story work can be done in a person's home and/or in supported living environments, such as in a care home, and there is no time limit on how long such a life story should take to work through. Importantly, as Kate Gridley and her colleagues have recently argued in a major UK-based study on life story work and practices, there is no one 'correct' way to develop a life story, and it is often a highly individualised activity that can take many forms (Gridley, Birks and Parker 2020). For example, some families, people with dementia and care practitioners work together to develop a chronological life story book that starts with the person's childhood and moves forward via major life milestones and events, such as teenage years, favourite holidays and so forth, and on to the present day. These life story books are often supported by photographs and other personal mementos from the person's life to help give additional insight and awareness in the storytelling. In contrast, other families/ people with dementia/care practitioners may take a more structured approach and follow a life story template which can be downloaded for free from the internet (see 'Resources and further reading' at the end of this chapter). However, no matter how it is tackled, the compilation and use of a life story enables the person with dementia to remain at the forefront of their life experiences, choices and values. Furthermore, a well-developed life story will also help to initiate and sustain interaction for and by the person with dementia by giving others key insights from which to develop meaningful communication approaches, such as by the undertaking of reminiscence work and/or creative art practices.

Returning to Surinder's text, the shared narrative also reveals that a life story is not a static object: it is a living document and record and a sensory connection to the outside world. Towards the end of her narrative, Surinder describes moving beyond the collation of her mother's life story and into the generation of life story as a *product* that could stand as a testimony to Bibi's life, memories and standing in the family. As Surinder shared in her writing, the breadth, depth and connectivity of Bibi's presented life story evolved when other family members also started to participate in its construction – for instance, by converting old VHS tapes to a CD format, enhancing the life story with the use of Punjabi books of short stories for Bibi to read, and by providing a repository of Bibi's favourite films on DVD so that they could be watched in either the here and now or in the times to come. Arguably, this enhancement to Bibi's life story was not undertaken as a task to be performed to enable person-centred care to take place, but instead as an expression of family love and gratitude and as a way to keep their mother's identity alive and ever present. This collective and creative action is also a lesson for practice. The task is not simply to collate and produce the life story of a person with dementia, however important that may be, but to actively use and apply it in an everyday context for the wellbeing of that person.

Reflecting on the above, this development and forward-thinking use of life story work by Surinder and her family is very much in the spirit of what Gridley *et al.* (2020), after consulting with various stakeholder groups, including family carers and people with dementia, put forward as 'good practice in life story work'. Here, the authors suggested that such good practice should: be tailored to the individual needs and preferences of the person with dementia; recognise that not everyone will want to take part in life story work and that some people may even find it distressing; be led by the person with dementia themselves; recognise the need for training and support for staff, caregivers and volunteers; include the potential for life story work to celebrate the person's life today and look to the future (Gridley *et al.* 2020, p.191). In many ways, Surinder's narrative and the co-production of Bibi's life story with her family are a testimony to what is good practice in life story work as identified by the research literature and stand as an outstanding example of person-centred care practices. In taking forward life story work, we can all learn from the words, experiences, wisdom and actions of Surinder and her family.

ADMIRAL NURSE ADVICE

Nikki Rowe, Admiral Nurse, The Orders of St John Care Trust

I am often asked by families about life stories and how best to develop them. This can include the most appropriate format for their life story but also helping them to think about which way is best for the person with dementia and their family. When creating a life story, the ideal is to start as soon as possible after a diagnosis of dementia to ensure full participation of the person with dementia; it is *their* life story after all.

This makes the life story more likely to reflect the person's wishes and preferences and encourages a sense of participation and ownership. Talk and plan the life story together, offering help and guidance where needed. How the life story information is collected is very individual. It can be written or be voice or visually recorded, as in Surinder and Bibi's case. It can sometimes be a combination of all of these. Seeing the story unfold at the point of recording can have a powerful effect on both the person with dementia and family members, as we see when Bibi talks of her experiences of Partition. So, as you see, there are many options for how you format a life story, and it's purely about which suits you both. Here are a few examples:

- **A scrapbook**

  This is a really nice way to document stories of life and add things such as photos or recipes – anything that is meaningful to that person. If you are artistic, you can scribble and draw, which adds to the personalisation of the scrapbook. Yes, this may look scruffy over time, but this can also become part of its 'loved' look.

- **Photo album**

  A photo album is an instantly recognisable and very traditional way to represent a life story. Most people will have photo albums in their house from which to develop a life story. You could add the names of people in the photos, the year it was taken, the event (perhaps a wedding or seaside holiday) and perhaps the relationship of people in the photo to the person with dementia. This may help later in orientation. You can also buy talking photo albums in which you can prerecord your voice, so when the person with dementia looks at a photo, they will hear you saying who it is or what the occasion was. This is a great way to enable the person with dementia to connect with both the image and your voice.

- **An auditory life story**

  An auditory life story can be a collection of songs and music that has specific meaning to the person with dementia over time, such as their own 'Top 10' songs they sang as a child or danced to as a teenager. Some people prefer listening rather than looking for the format of a life story. Listening to an auditory life story can be done while walking and often can be of value at times of distress or ill-being (see Purple Angel's MP3 Players in the 'Resources and further reading' section at the end of this chapter).

- **Collage**

  Life story can be captured as a collage and displayed on a wall. It is a very visual format of life story and effective for someone with dementia who is less mobile or in bed. The collage could be of photos, brief narrative and stories, specific memories, postcards, tickets – in fact, anything that has a significance to that person. In Bibi's case, a collage may include a map of the region in India where Bibi lived, photos of milking the cows, perhaps a recipe for samosas, or even cotton reels to depict when Bibi worked as a machinist. Collages can be a very creative approach to life story.

- **Memory box/rummage box**

  Similar to a collage, a memory or rummage box is a collection of important things representative of a person life but kept in a box rather than on the wall. Memory boxes are quite tactile and can be a very enjoyable and exploratory experience each time a person with dementia delves into it.

Any of the above suggestions can be interchanged and used at different stages of the dementia journey. It may be, as the person's condition changes, that you feel the introduction of a different life story format would be helpful.

When can a life story be used?

Life stories can be brought into use on many occasions. For example, when a person with dementia is feeling anxious or low about their dementia, a life story may enable them to focus on positive aspects of their life rather than dwell on negative feelings. Where possible, make this as relaxing as you can, perhaps accompanied by a sociable drink, such as a cup of tea.

A life story can be an effective way of connecting with the person with dementia, especially if they are feeling disorientated, distressed or anxious. It can also assist a family member to feel part of *their* world and meet them where *they* are, as opposed to trying to get them to fit into ours.

It may seem repetitive for you to use their life story with the person with dementia again and again. However, it is important to consider that if some benefit and wellbeing is achieved, then it does not matter how often the story is revisited. For the person with dementia, telling the story and reliving those emotional memories is the key and likely to engender a sense of accomplishment and usefulness.

The compilation of a life story is continuous and potentially never ends as it can carry on as part of a wider family story, as a legacy of the life of the person with dementia. It can be useful to encourage wider family members to get involved as the person with dementia may recount and recall different things with different family members influenced by their relationship to them. This will make a well-rounded life story.

REFERENCES

Gridley, K., Birks, Y. and Parker, G. (2020) 'Exploring good practice in life story work with people with dementia: The findings of a qualitative study looking at the multiple views of stakeholders.' *Dementia 19*, 2, 182–194.

Kitwood, T. (1997) *Dementia Reconsidered: The Person Comes First*. Buckingham: Open University Press.

RESOURCES AND FURTHER READING

Gridley, K., Brooks, J., Birks, Y., Baxter, K. and Parker, G. (2016) 'Improving care for people with dementia: Development and initial feasibility study for evaluation of life story work in dementia care.' *National Institute of Health Research, Health Services and Delivery Research 4*, 23. doi:10.3310/hsdr04230.

Kindell, J., Burrow, S., Wilkinson, R. and Keady, J.D. (2014) 'Life story resources in dementia care: A review.' *Quality in Ageing and Older Adults 15*, 3, 151–161. doi:10.1108/QAOA-02-2014-0003.

Dementia UK
CREATING A LIFE STORY

www.dementiauk.org/?s=Life+story

Purple Angel's MP3 Players

The purpose of the Purple Angel Dementia Campaign is to raise awareness, give hope to and empower people with dementia by providing information on how shops, businesses and other services can support people who have these progressive diseases – both elderly and younger onset. They also provide free bespoke MP3 players to people with dementia.

https://purpleangelcornwall.weebly.com/mp3-players-and-music-for-dementia.html

CHAPTER 2

'I kept telling myself that he was still grieving for Mum'

DIAGNOSING DEMENTIA IN LATER LIFE

Molly Barry (pseudonym)

My parents were devoted to each other, although everyone considered them the most unlikely of pairings. My mum was a quiet and private person while my dad was loud and outgoing with a mischievous streak – Mum called him a loveable rogue. They moved about 30 miles away from my brother and me when they retired to be near the sea. We were a close family and saw each other as much as we could. About three and a half years ago, Mum had said to me that Dad 'wasn't himself'. When I asked her what she meant, she said, 'I am not sure but something's different.' As time passed, she felt that he had 'lost his sparkle', but when we visited, Dad seemed as jovial as ever, cracking jokes and making a fuss of the grandchildren. I suggested to Mum that maybe he was in pain as he had needed two knee replacements since before he retired, and he was now 79 but he still refused to do anything about it. Mum smiled and said, no matter what, he wouldn't go to the GP and, anyway, perhaps it was just a part of getting older. She never spoke about it again.

A year ago, Mum died suddenly following a brain haemorrhage. She was in the garden and collapsed. She never regained consciousness. Dad went to the hospital with her and was with her when she died. We were all devastated. At that point, I wished Dad lived even closer to me so I could keep an eye on him, but he said he wanted to stay put as it had been their forever home. My brother and I and the older grandchildren made sure we regularly visited and checked on him. He seemed to be doing OK, although we did notice he was losing weight. We thought that might be because Mum had always been a great cook and would always load up your plate. As the weeks passed, Dad's mood seemed to dip; he was less chatty and would cut phone calls short with an excuse that he was about to go out. Sometimes when we visited, he would not be there, which was not like him, and the house was getting really untidy. I told Dad I was worried about him and thought he should go to the GP for a check-up. Although he was not keen, he said he would make an appointment. I also suggested we get him someone in to help with the cleaning as that had always been Mum's domain. He became cross and said he didn't need any help and was happy as he was.

I asked him how he got on at the GP and he said that he had got some tablets and he was feeling much better. I was relieved and didn't pry further as he didn't like to talk about things like that. About six months after Mum died, I started getting calls from Dad late at night saying he couldn't find Mum and he was worried. I had to keep reminding him that Mum was dead and that he had been with her at the end. He would say, 'Of course she died; I must have fallen asleep in the chair again and forgotten where I was.' Then last Christmas happened. Dad came to stay with us as I didn't want him to be on his own at Christmas. Dad had never stayed at ours before. I was surprised that he hadn't packed many things to bring with him, and when I asked if he needed anything else, he snapped at me. Dad never usually snapped at anyone, and I was more shocked when he didn't seem bothered that had I started to cry. Over Christmas, he wore the same clothes every day and didn't have a shower or a bath. He slept most of the day and was up and down all night, and he barely ate a thing. He wasn't like my dad at all. I kept telling myself that he was still grieving for Mum, but my husband said, 'Do you think that it could be more than that?' I asked him what he meant, and he said, 'Do you think your dad has got dementia?' In our culture, dementia is something that is not talked about as there is still so much stigma and discrimination, so I was furious that he could suggest such a thing and walked away from the conversation.

Dad had a fall the day after Boxing Day and was taken to hospital. They found he had a urine infection, and he was admitted. He was really confused and aggressive towards the nursing staff. They asked my brother and me if he had been experiencing any problems before the infection. I told them that he had been to the GP a couple of months ago and got some tablets but didn't know what they were for. They checked with the GP surgery who confirmed that he did make an appointment but never attended. They added that there had been several calls from my mum before she died, saying she was worried about his behaviour, and although she had tried to get him to see the GP, he refused to go. They said he had not collected his prescription for pain medication for several months either. I was shocked. I felt terrible that I had let him and my mum down.

The hospital doctors requested a CT scan and said they thought he might have vascular dementia but would ask someone to review him after he was discharged from hospital to give him time to recover from the infection. Dad wasn't able to go home because he was too confused; he went to a residential care home near where I live. A nurse from the local memory assessment team came to assess him a few weeks later in the care home and said he had vascular dementia, that it was quite advanced and there was nothing that could be done. I still feel angry, guilty and confused. I wish I had listened to my mum; I wish I had seen what was happening and maybe things would have been different for all of us.

SPECIALIST COMMENTARY

Manisha Ray, Consultant Old Age Psychiatrist, Nottinghamshire Healthcare NHS Foundation Trust

Dementia is a debilitating progressive illness that affects several areas of brain function. The commonest early symptoms of dementia are memory problems (e.g. forgetfulness, not remembering recent information, losing everyday objects more often), difficulties in thinking through and organising tasks (e.g. managing finances, managing property), impaired problem solving (e.g. coming up with ideas, solutions when faced with challenges), difficulties in completing tasks that require following instructions in multiple steps (e.g. following a recipe to prepare fresh meals), language difficulties (e.g. slow speech, word-finding difficulties), poor orientation (e.g. not finding way back even in familiar places), visuospatial difficulties (e.g. not being able to assess things in three dimensions such as height of stairs) and changes in mood and emotions (irritability, low mood, anxiety, mood swings). The presentation might vary depending on type of dementia. Memory problems are more prominent in Alzheimer's dementia than other types. In vascular dementia, non-memory symptoms, such as planning and organising tasks, problem solving, judgement and visuospatial ability, may be affected early on.

Diagnosis of dementia may be delayed due to the family not recognising or seeking advice about the changes they observe. Sometimes it is difficult to recognise that the observed changes may need attention. In the above case discussion, Molly's mother was the first person to raise suspicion about her husband's change of personality ('something's different', 'lost his sparkle'). However, other family members couldn't see it when they saw her father. Gradual onset and variable symptoms at the early stage make it difficult for others to identify an onset of possible dementia. The individual with dementia often lacks insight into their difficulties. Lack of insight delays and sometimes can interfere with seeking help even if their spouse or other family members identify difficulties. Due to its slow progression, the immediate family member living with the individual (e.g. partner) sometimes gradually and unknowingly takes on several household responsibilities, compensating for the person's difficulties. The problems are detected only when there is a breakdown in this support system. In Molly's father's case, it was only recognised he was having problems when Molly's mother died.

Lack of awareness about dementia and its early signs among individuals and family members also contributes to missing the mild symptoms at an earlier stage. In general, public perception of dementia is associated only with memory problems, and other non-memory cognitive symptoms may be overlooked. Had Molly's mother and other family members had more awareness and psychoeducation on dementia, they could have identified and articulated the problems earlier to seek appropriate help from the services. Misinformation and societal attitudes towards normal ageing, e.g. that memory impairment is an inevitable part of growing old, also act to delay seeking help and accessing services.

Comorbid physical and mental health issues can make it more difficult to detect early signs of dementia. For example, it is hard to identify additional cognitive and functional deficits in people with existing deficits, for example, due to stroke or Parkinson's disease. Additional psychological factors such as depression or bereavement can cause difficulties in identifying symptoms of dementia as they can often present in similar fashion. In Molly's father's case, complicating factors including the practical implications of his wife's absence (no cooked meals) and the psychological impact of her loss (grief) clouded Molly's understanding of her father's presentation. Detection of dementia could take longer in people who live alone and have little or no contact with friends or family. Their cognitive deficits often come to the attention of services following incidents such as a fall, leaving the home at an unsociable hour or a house fire.

Socio-cultural factors such as stigma, shame, ethnicity and language barriers and unhelpful beliefs (e.g. nothing can be done) associated with dementia can also contribute to a delay in seeking help for family members. In Molly's case, she was angry when her husband suggested the possibility of dementia. Studies suggest that people from minority ethnic backgrounds seek help for dementia diagnosis and care later than the majority of the population. Beliefs about the cause of cognitive impairment, negative beliefs about psychiatry and a sense of family responsibilities are potential barriers in seeking diagnosis of dementia at an early stage (Mukadam, Cooper and Livingston 2011). Other studies show negative beliefs about the benefits of a diagnosis and treatment in South Asian communities, which affects their willingness to seek help. Dementia disproportionately affects Black African and Caribbean communities as compared with other ethnic minorities and the majority population. Despite having a higher dementia risk, black older adults are less likely to get a timely diagnosis or receive treatment and support for dementia. Beliefs such as dementia doesn't affect black people, negative experience of health and social care services, beliefs around kinship and familial responsibility, and religious and spiritual beliefs were found to be contributing to delay in help seeking for people of Black African and Caribbean ethnicity in the UK.

In the UK, primary care professionals play a crucial role in identifying signs of dementia, triggering referral to secondary services for confirmation of diagnosis. Clinicians at the primary care level need to be familiar with warning signs that may indicate suspected dementia, such as missed appointments, issues around taking medications and family carers raising concerns to the primary care professionals. Studies of primary care have highlighted several factors that can contribute to delayed or missed diagnosis. Such factors may include variation in skills of diagnosis and management of dementia, challenges around balancing pressure on time, inadequate access and communication with specialist services and social care, and concerns about negative impact of the diagnostic label of dementia on patients and family.

In Molly's father's case, he had missed his appointment with his GP and did not collect his prescription medications for several months. Her mother had called the GP's surgery several times before she died, expressing concern about her husband's behaviour and refusal to attend appointments.

Over the last few years, there has been some improvement in the public's awareness of dementia due to media coverage and initiatives such as Dementia Friends and dementia-friendly communities. However, some communities still fear the stigma and discrimination of the diagnosis. Usually, immediate family members first recognise the early signs of dementia. They then approach other family, friends or health professionals about their worries. Recent policies and guidance have promoted the early detection and diagnosis of dementia and advocated the benefits of this for the person with dementia and their family. This has had led to some improvement in the diagnosis rate of dementia, but more needs to be done to improve this further.

ADMIRAL NURSE ADVICE

Stuart Kennedy, Admiral Nurse and Independent Prescriber, Charnwood GP Network

Getting a diagnosis
Going to the GP for regular check-ups can help identify changes to an older person's usual presentation, such as their mood, personality and appearance. Often the GP will invite the person in for a health check or medication review and include screening tests such as blood

tests to rule out any potentially treatable cause of the changes. If all physical or psychological conditions have been ruled out, the GP may refer the person for further investigation to a memory assessment clinic or specialist.

Primary care staff may undertake memory-screening tests at a person's annual health check, and this can be a useful opportunity to identify changes to memory early on and discuss what happens next. As Dr Ray highlights, skills among primary care staff may vary in being able to recognise worrying signs. Opportunities to observe for any changes exist within primary care when annually reviewing patients with other co-morbidities, such as diabetes. A proactive approach should focus on asking the patient to consent to a memory test rather than asking 'Are you worried about your memory?' which may miss those who lack insight.

Families should be prepared for the likely pathway before any referral to memory assessment services is made. Once GPs have routinely conducted blood tests to ensure any treatable causes of changes to memory are identified and corrected, discussions may follow around other potential causes. Such changes in a person may be the beginning of dementia but may also indicate untreated depression or other underlying health conditions. GPs will discuss treating such conditions and reviewing the person again in 1–2 months to see if there is an improvement. If there is no change, a referral for a memory assessment will usually follow.

The assessment process

When a referral is received by a memory assessment clinic, they will allocate it to the most appropriate professional to see the person based upon the information they receive and arrange an appointment (how this is conducted will vary from clinic to clinic while the effects of COVID-19 require continued social distancing). Often the memory assessment clinic may request a scan of the person's brain to assist in a diagnosis; however, undertaking this type of test will vary across clinics depending on the person's age and whether or not their presentation is considered atypical (i.e. one that is unusual). During the appointment, a member of clinic staff will record information about the person: their personal background, medical and psychiatric history, normal personality, duration of symptoms, self-care abilities, sleep, mood and any other information that will assist with an accurate diagnosis.

It is usual to conduct a detailed memory test to provide much more information on key areas including memory, concentration, word finding, comprehension and visuospatial abilities. Once the assessment has been completed, the results are often discussed with other professionals in the team to affirm findings and/or consider any further tests or assessments. The person will be offered a follow-up appointment where the results of all assessment tests will be discussed and, if appropriate, a diagnosis will be made and any potential interventions and treatments discussed. The appointment where the diagnosis of dementia is given can feel overwhelming for the person with dementia and their family. There is a lot of information to take in and many are not prepared or know what to ask. It is important that family members are prepared for the possibility of the diagnosis of dementia and give thought to how this might change things for each of them.

A diagnosis should not just be about giving a name to explain the problems experienced, but should be an opportunity to offer tailored advice and information. In some types of dementia, such as Alzheimer's disease or mixed dementia (commonly Alzheimer's and vascular), medications, such as donepezil, may be prescribed by the memory assessment clinic. Where the type of dementia does not respond to this medication, it is common for there to be no further follow-up beyond this point. The person being offered medication must be able to understand the risks and benefits of treatment and weigh these up (this is referred to as mental capacity and is assessed on each separate decision). Where the person cannot, it would not be common for treatment to be offered without a very strong case of it being in the person's best interest.

Involvement in future research may also be discussed, as the quest to identify improved treatments and care continues apace. This may involve discussion of a local study or larger-scale studies over various centres, but in both cases agreement to be contacted by researchers and added to a database is sought first.

As you can see, there is a lot to be discussed at a diagnosis appointment, so it is often useful to go prepared with specific questions and perhaps have these written down to prompt you to ask. In the case of Molly's father, the lack of an early diagnosis limited the extent of advice and interventions that could be given to Molly's father, and the family, about how to prevent further vascular damage to the brain (e.g. managing vascular issues such as high blood pressure and/or cholesterol levels, dietary changes, reducing lifestyle risks). It also limited the family's discussion about plans for the future and support packages that could have helped him to stay at home longer.

Molly's story

As we see in the case of Molly and her parents, many families can face significant obstacles in getting a timely diagnosis of dementia. As explored in the specialist section, many factors can contribute to this, and where stigma or poor awareness of the condition exists, a diagnosis may be delayed by months or even years. Molly's father did not visit the GP and so this opportunity was missed.

When thinking about early signs, it is important to ensure that poor hearing and/or eyesight are not hindering a person's communication and conveying an appearance of forgetfulness. It can be valuable for families to have a broad idea of some symptoms that might be a concern and prompt discussion with the GP. As Dr Ray details, there are several common and early signs that may lead the person and/or their families to be concerned. Molly's mother recognised that something wasn't quite right and tried to discuss her concerns with the GP, but her husband did not attend the appointments.

A visit to the GP may be avoided for several reasons, such as not wanting to bother the GP as they believe what they are experiencing is a normal part of ageing and not being aware of how the changes are having an impact on their life (managing appointments, medication, driving, etc.). Many, however, may refuse to attend due to a fear of dementia and how this may affect their life. It is important to reassure the person that their symptoms need investigating as there are many physical health and psychological conditions that mimic dementia, and these may be treatable. However, a refusal to go to the GP, for whatever reason, can cause frustration and distress within the family. In these cases, the family should seek advice on what to do next. Molly explains the changes in personality she had noticed (being uncharacteristically snappy), alongside the sense of dementia not being commonly talked about in her culture. Undoubtedly, such stigma can lead to unfortunate delays in accessing the right support.

The Admiral Nurse role

Admiral Nurses support people throughout the journey with dementia, from conversations leading to assessment and diagnosis to support and advice to families following diagnosis.

Admiral Nurses work closely with colleagues in primary care to promote screening for dementia, encourage early recognition and support best practice by promoting wider awareness of early signs. If situations alter, the Admiral Nurse can liaise with memory clinic colleagues to ensure referrals are regularly discussed and seen sooner, where required. Following a diagnosis, Admiral Nurses can assist with very practical issues such as applying for benefits (e.g. attendance allowance and council tax reduction), talking through legal aspects (e.g. Lasting Power of Attorney, Tenancy in Common) and any issues that the family are finding it difficult to understand or adapt to. There may be many questions within families around what to expect in the future, how to respond to particular symptoms and how to access wider community support.

As the condition progresses, families may also need advice on how to manage issues such as driving, managing finances and how to respond to symptoms. Discussions about driving, and whether to cease or not at this point, can sometimes be difficult for the person with dementia to accept. The memory assessment clinic will have a legal obligation to advise someone to stop driving straight away if they feel they are unsafe, but this is uncommon. In most cases, the person and/or family will be instructed to inform DVLA (Driver and Vehicle Licensing Agency) and motor insurer of the diagnosis, so that annual reviews of safety can be arranged. In some cases, the person with dementia may be directed to take an on-the-road test locally to determine safety.

The support before and following diagnosis is central in ensuring families are able to seek advice, ask questions and access support and care as and when they most need it to ensure they are not left feeling alone.

REFERENCES

Mukadam, N., Cooper, C. and Livingston, G. (2011) 'A systematic review of ethnicity and pathways to care in dementia.' *International Journal of Geriatric Psychiatry 26*, 1, 12–20. doi:10.1002/gps.2484.

RESOURCES AND FURTHER READING
What to expect at diagnosis

www.nice.org.uk/about/nice-communities/social-care/quick-guides/
dementia-discussing-and-planning-support-after-diagnosis

After diagnosis of dementia: what to expect from health and social care services

www.gov.uk/government/publications/after-a-diagnosis-of-
dementia-what-to-expect-from-health-and-care-services/
after-diagnosis-of-dementia-what-to-expect-from-health-and-care-
services

Dementia UK
HOW TO GET A DIAGNOSIS OF DEMENTIA

www.dementiauk.org/get-support/diagnosis-and-specialist-
suppport/getting-a-diagnosis-of-dementia

AFTER A DIAGNOSIS: NEXT STEPS CHECKLIST

www.dementiauk.org/get-support/diagnosis-and-specialist-
suppport/after-a-diagnosis-of-dementia-next-steps-checklist

PRACTICAL GUIDE TO GETTING THE BEST OUT
OF GP AND OTHER HEALTH APPOINTMENTS

www.dementiauk.org/get-support/diagnosis-and-specialist-
suppport/practical-guide-to-getting-the-best-out-of-gp-and-other-
health-appointments

CHAPTER 3

'Getting a diagnosis is not easy'

DIAGNOSING DEMENTIA IN YOUNGER ADULTS

Rob Garrett

Jayne, my partner, was involved in a road traffic collision with a lorry seven years ago. Fortunately, she was not physically injured, but it was still a very traumatic experience, and she didn't drive or work after this. It may have been coincidental, but we then noticed subtle changes in Jayne's cognitive abilities, which we thought were due to post-traumatic stress. I tried to get Jayne to seek help, but she flatly refused, in her normal feisty, independent manner.

Over the next two years, I noticed that her memory and recall deteriorated, and, strangely, her eyesight. The first indication of her deteriorating memory was when she rang me during her usual morning walk, to say she couldn't remember her way back to the path leading down into town. At the same time, I also noticed that Jayne's walking pace had become slow and tentative on rough terrain. The changes in her vision became evident when she seemed unable to sow seeds in our allotment and lost interest in reading, which was out of character. She was a frequent user of our local library. Jayne had always had regular eye tests because of her diabetes but now became flustered and struggled with the test. She had prescription glasses but never really used them, saying they didn't 'feel right', and she was confused between the reading and distance pairs.

I was made redundant, but despite being offered a similar position, I turned it down as I was becoming increasingly concerned about Jayne. I decided to take some time out, as I needed to be closer to home. Things settled for a while, so I started a part-time job from 5am to 10am, which allowed me to be with Jayne during the day. I would sleep downstairs, getting up at 4am, have some cereal, which I would lay out the previous night. One morning, my breakfast had been eaten. I joked with Jayne about it later, but she had no clue what I was talking about. From that point, Jayne's sleep became more disturbed, for which she saw an acupuncturist as she did not want to take medications. That night, Jayne experienced the most frightening and vivid nightmare with hallucinations, and from then her sleep deteriorated even more. It was not long after this that Jayne fainted during one of our walks. Jayne refused to see her GP, but a few weeks later she had several fainting episodes in succession, whereupon I called an ambulance. The paramedics said Jayne's blood pressure had dropped. She did then agree to see her GP who took some blood tests, but no further investigations seemed to follow. She didn't want to mention anything about her memory problems. There were a few more visits to the GP following this, but nothing was followed up. It was mainly a chat about Jayne's overall health, with little input from Jayne.

Jayne's behaviour started to include sundowning (see Chapter 13), and her vision and spatial awareness deteriorated even more. She now struggled to make a cup of tea, use the cooker or make a sandwich. At this time, she also began having false beliefs, wanting to 'go home' (even though she was at home), and at one point, Jayne thought I was an imposter, which I now know is called Capgras syndrome. One of our sons took her to the GP but was advised that unless Jayne admitted to the problems herself, there was nothing the GP could do. I changed my shift patterns to be with her more, and family filled the gaps; if left alone, Jayne would become very confused, which was noticed by our neighbours. We continued to go for short walks and work the allotment, but even this was becoming more difficult. Although the allotment was behind our house, Jayne did not have the confidence to go alone.

That same year, Jayne went into hospital for successive faints, which continued even while in the accident and emergency department. She was only in hospital for a brief period, but there was noticeable deterioration when back home. Jayne believed that small flecks of dust or dirt were insects, and her walking pace or gait slowed even more. She found it almost impossible to walk outside in the dark. Jayne now struggled with steps, requiring help to get up and down, but the most noticeable change was that Jayne could not remember how to use the toilet – not seeming to see it or know where to sit. I changed the seat to a strong colour, but this only made her more anxious about using it. During the hospital admission, the clinical team were focused on the cause of her problems being organic or reversible, despite CT and MRI head scans both showing marked brain atrophy. During the ward rounds, the clinicians and consultants confirmed chronic progressive cognitive impairment. Jayne was discharged two days later with a follow-up appointment. The discharge notes said I would need support in my caring role, but this never happened. We saw the neurologist for follow-up early the next year, and he undertook various practical tests and said he thought Jayne was showing symptoms of Parkinsonism and wanted to refer her for a DaT scan. Suggesting this made Jayne's anxiety increase to a level I've never seen before. She was frightened and refused the DaT scan, and any mention of the doctor's name after that would generate anxiety and panic. The neurologist was still unclear as to the cause of Jayne's symptoms and mentioned terms such as corticobasal degeneration and posterior cortical atrophy. This was a foreign language to me, but at no point did he mention dementia.

I was frustrated, as I knew that Jayne was living with it. We came away with a diagnosis of non-specific cognitive impairment. We then had a period of stability, but it didn't last. She started to become extremely angry and swore, which was out of character, and her senses seemed heightened. Sometimes I had to whisper as she said I spoke too loudly, or when I cuddled her, she said my arm was heavy and hurt. She experienced more hallucinations and the Capgras worsened. She often thought she could feel water spraying on her and eventually became reluctant to shower. As Jayne's condition worsened, I knew this was dementia, not Jayne.

Four years later, Jayne was referred to the memory clinic for an assessment. I didn't tell her this was where we were going for fear she wouldn't go. Visits to the GP had already proved fruitless. It was when a referral was made to the local depression and anxiety service that I realised the GP wasn't quite sure what to do. At that same time, the neurologist wanted to see Jayne, but I knew she wouldn't go. I tried everything, even asking if it was possible to see a female neurologist.

What helped move things along was when I managed to get both Jayne and me registered with the same GP, and it was then we managed to get a female neurologist involved. However, throughout the appointment Jayne kept saying she was OK, she was managing fine, doing the housework, and apart from her diabetes, nothing was wrong with her. I felt very frustrated, and indeed angry, as I felt this may also be a missed opportunity. After the appointment, the neurologist wrote a letter suggesting a DaT scan, should Jayne wish to go! Was no one listening to what I had to say? The letter also suggested the next step would be a formal assessment of her capacity, and after this, carry things out on a best interest basis, and whether Jayne could be given the diagnosis of dementia. In the meantime, I hoped Jayne would agree to a DaT scan.

This was now beginning to affect me and my mental state. As I witnessed the rapid deterioration, the delusions, false beliefs, hallucinations, everything seemed to be ignored or not taken seriously. Within two weeks of this appointment, Jayne was again admitted to hospital, this time to a psychiatric hospital. After a very long and torturous journey of over seven years, a diagnosis of Alzheimer's or dementia with Lewy bodies was now mooted.

SPECIALIST COMMENTARY

Dr Jacqui Hussey, Consultant Old Age Psychiatrist and Lead Consultant for the Memory Clinic in Wokingham, Berkshire Healthcare Trust

Young-onset dementia, defined as dementia under the age of 65, can present many challenges to diagnosis. There are an estimated 42,325 people with young-onset dementia in the UK (Alzheimer's Society 2014) but traditional dementia diagnostic and support services are primarily aimed at older people. Timely diagnosis is essential to access the support needed to adapt to life with young-onset dementia and to lower carer stress levels (Bakker *et al.* 2010; Carter, Oyebode and Koopmans 2017).

The different needs of people with young-onset dementia

Developing dementia at a younger age can bring about specific problems. People almost inevitably reduce their working hours or give up employment, with consequent financial concerns as they may still have a mortgage and dependent children. In addition, there are psychological, social and relationship implications for both the person with young-onset dementia and their partner, which are different from those diagnosed with dementia at an older age. The Needs in Young Onset Dementia (NeedYD) study found that younger people with dementia have high levels of unmet needs with respect to activity engagement, socialisation, intimate relationships, psychological distress and information. This increases the risk of behavioural and psychological symptoms of dementia such as agitation and low mood (Bakker *et al.* 2010).

The Angela Project undertook an England-wide survey and made key recommendations for best practice for people with young-onset dementia which included providing access to young-onset-specific information and support, supported age-appropriate activity and support to maintain physical and mental health as well as possible (Stamou *et al.* 2019).

Delays to a diagnosis

The INSPIRED study showed that on average it took 3.2 years to diagnosis for someone with young-onset dementia and up to 4.7 years to being told which subtype of dementia they had (Draper *et al.* 2016).

Jayne and Rob's story highlights many of the difficulties people with young-onset dementia experience. First, there is often a lack of recognition that someone under the age of 65, sometimes in their 30s, 40s or 50s, can get dementia. For the layperson, the term 'dementia' is often associated with ageing, senility and frailty. Similarly, for GPs and healthcare professionals, dementia in a younger person is often not on their radar or is low down on a list of many other possible diagnoses. It is not uncommon for early symptoms to be attributed to anxiety or post-traumatic stress disorder, as in Jayne's case, or to be misdiagnosed as depression or other psychiatric illness.

Additionally, people may be reluctant to seek help. They may be unaware of some of their cognitive difficulties or do not wish to acknowledge them because of fear of the future, concerns about the impact on the relationship with their partner and other family members, or even a belief that there is nothing that can be done. Denial mechanisms can protect an individual from anxiety about their illness. The fact that Jayne 'flatly refused' suggests that she was in denial about her symptoms. Although it may be thought that denial mechanisms (anosognosia – a lack of insight) in dementia may protect an individual from anxiety about their illness, this did not seem to be the case for Jayne. Contact with her GP at this stage could have provided Jayne and Rob with the opportunity for pre-diagnostic counselling.

Diagnostic complexity

Younger people are more likely to present with atypical symptoms and/or have a rarer form of dementia. As a result, GPs are often uncertain about where to refer younger people with suspected dementia and, furthermore, there are few designated services in the UK that are commissioned to provide young-onset diagnostic services and age-appropriate aftercare.

In an older person, dementia-type symptoms are more likely to be due to dementia (see Chapter 2), but in a younger person it is even more essential not to miss so-called 'reversible' causes of cognitive symptoms, which may have the effect of extending the investigation period. When cognitive difficulties arise at a younger age, it is important to rule out autoimmune, metabolic and genetic causes. Rarer conditions such as posterior cortical atrophy, frontotemporal dementia and language-variant dementia, and the so-called Parkinson-Plus conditions such as corticobasal degeneration, should always be considered. Eighty per cent of people present with non-cognitive symptoms. Consequently, without a coordinated referral pathway, people are variously referred to neurology, rheumatology, opticians, mental health services and memory clinics.

When eventually conditions such as posterior cortical atrophy and corticobasal degeneration were suggested to Rob and Jayne, they were not given any explanation that these diseases are subtypes of dementia. The Angela Project (Stamou *et al.* 2019) reported that the experience of receiving a diagnosis could be improved through clinicians' use of language.

The pursuit of a diagnosis subtype is understandable and expected. However, the lack of a coordinated referral pathway and joined-up services to achieve this, and a less than pragmatic approach in Jayne's case, left Rob with little understanding of Jayne's symptoms, unable to access appropriate support and validation, and, importantly, no knowing how to cope. Unfortunately, this is a common experience for family carers of younger people with dementia.

Carer's perspective

When dementia occurs at an early age, the psychological and social implications for both people with dementia and their family carers are numerous. They are in a phase of their life when they would normally play an active role in employment and family life. Fifty per cent of partners of a person with dementia give up work, and this can lead to mood changes, carer stress and isolation. Lack of support and information about the diagnosis and treatment approaches can make a lonely experience even more isolating. It is also worth remembering that the family carer of someone with young-onset dementia may also be their child or their parent.

In the early stages, Jayne was reluctant to seek help, and both Rob and professionals wished to respect her autonomy and preferences. Nevertheless, throughout the course of her illness, Jayne's mental capacity needed to be assessed and reassessed. If she lacked under-standing or insight into her illness, there were still opportunities to address specific symptoms of dementia, such as her sleep disturbance and delusional thinking, independently of a diagnosis being reached. Rob, who had to reconfigure and reduce his working hours to become a full-time carer, would have benefited from education and support. This could have improved both Jayne and Rob's wellbeing.

Family carers surveyed in the Angela Project (Stamou *et al.* 2019) reported that they wanted information specific to young-onset dementia and targeted advice on how to cope, and support to con-tinue their life outside of their caring role, such as having employment and to feel connected. In Rob's case, the long and frustrating path to Jayne's diagnosis of dementia, coupled with his anxiety and lack of awareness about what help was available, denied him all of these.

What supports might have helped?

It is important for family carers to be offered support in their own right and to be referred to social care for a carer's assessment. Knowledge and education about Jayne's symptom clusters could have helped Rob and other family members to continue to support Jayne. Rob could have benefited through signposting to local supports such as a Dementia Care Advisor or Admiral Nursing service. He could also have been given information about, for example: financial benefits (which are different for people under 65), Lasting Power of Attorney, local charity support, and national organisations such as the Alzheimer's Society and Dementia UK which hosts the Young Dementia Network and Rare Dementia Support. With this specialist advice and support, Rob and Jayne's experience of living with the effects of young-onset dementia could have been very different.

ADMIRAL NURSE ADVICE

Fiona Chaabane, Consultant Admiral Nurse/ Clinical Nurse Specialist in Younger Onset Dementia and Huntington's Disease, University Hospital Southampton NHS Foundation Trust

Getting a diagnosis

It is probably fair to say that no one expects to be diagnosed with dementia at a young age.

The largest group affected by dementia is people aged over 65 years, and the prevalence and incidence increases as the decades pass (i.e. the percentage of people affected in their 80s is larger than those affected in their 70s). There are no sudden changes when we reach 65 years; this is merely an administrative demarcation that used to separate the working population from the retired population.

In dementia care, medical and social care services are focused on the area of most demand, the needs of older people. When a younger person is affected by dementia, they may find the services available are not age-appropriate, do not address their particular presentation or needs, and may be difficult to access. In addition, the clinical expertise required to investigate a younger person with cognitive problems may be more scarce and sometimes only in specialist centres. Ironically, therefore, specialist centres (cognitive neurology clinics) develop huge expertise in diagnosing dementia in younger people but may not be accessed in a timely fashion.

Changing cognitive function

Some changes in cognitive function (the way the brain works things out, the ability to remember, preserve new memories, process information, form judgements, rationalise and so on) affect us all as we age. We notice that we might not be as mentally sharp as we used to be, may need a little more time to do things that we used to do without any hesitation. This is normal ageing and occurs as a part of natural 'wear and tear' for most. However, for some, a sustained and progressive change in cognitive function may indicate an illness such as dementia. There are many causes for cognitive change, and a review by a GP will lead to investigation of that cause depending on their initial findings.

Prior to diagnosis, a younger person may notice difficulties coping with day-to-day life, often reporting problems managing at work, but they may put this down to being tired, stressed, over-burdened with responsibilities or feeling low in mood. The first line of investigation therefore is to check that the person is not suffering from a reversible condition such as anaemia, depression/low mood or an autoimmune condition or thyroid disorder that might lead to similar symptoms to those seen in dementia. Ironically, the younger the person at this time, the longer the list of disorders that could be the cause and which need to be excluded. This in part explains the longer length of time it often takes to reach a diagnosis in a younger person: there are more investigations to be carried out that might include a range of types of brain imaging (e.g. CT, MRI, SPECT or PET scans) and neuropsychological assessment (where a neuropsychologist assesses how the different brain regions function to aid diagnosis), and, for some, a lumbar puncture may be required. All of this takes time and may include attending hospital clinics that are not local or undergoing imaging and screening that is not available at most hospitals. It is this higher level of investigation and complexity that prolongs the time to diagnosis so often reported.

Younger-onset dementia can be difficult to spot for most and, in an age-group where dementia is not suspected, hard to contemplate as a possibility. Cognitive problems are common in day-to-day life, but what makes these experiences different is the context within which these difficulties sit and the length of time they are apparent. Ironically, dementia is usually slow to reveal itself, and what appear to be isolated incidences initially can increase in frequency, complexity and impact as time passes. Families often describe episodes of concern that may have occurred years before diagnosis that, at the time, seemed odd but inconsequential. It is only later, once the diagnosis is known, that these events gain more significance in retrospect.

Diagnosing younger-onset dementia is multi-dimensional – there is not one test that can absolutely confirm or exclude such a diagnosis. Accurate diagnosis depends on the outcome of screening, cognitive and physical assessment, investigations, the person's presentation, the family story and possession of the relevant clinical expertise. It is all of these aspects which, when collated, help to form the picture of a condition that, depending on the stage at which it is investigated, can reveal the diagnosis. Even before a diagnosis, cognitive change can have a huge effect on the person, family and work life, and impact on relationships, finances, responsibilities and roles. The affected person and all of those around them will need support to adapt to accommodate to the person's changing abilities and needs while investigation is taking place.

Jayne and Rob's story

In Jayne's case, her symptoms were attributed to the impact of an accident following which she experienced an element of post-traumatic stress disorder. This is a completely reasonable assumption to make under the circumstances – however, after a period of time in which there was no improvement and increasing concern about cognitive function, investigation into the cause of the increasing difficulties was essential. Treatment for low mood or anxiety is necessary to alleviate those symptoms but also to better judge the true picture of function without those symptoms masking abilities. When there is no response to treatment, however, it would be reasonable to suspect that something else may be the cause.

Posterior cortical atrophy (PCA) – much publicised by the author Terry Pratchett who developed PCA – is thought to be caused by either Alzheimer's disease pathology or Lewy body disease and reflects brain changes that start towards the back of the brain where visual processing takes place. Patients with PCA often report failing eyesight to an optician, which is not remedied by a new spectacle prescription. However, the changes are specific and include only being able to see particular colours, being unable to see things that are translucent (e.g. glass doors), having difficulty focusing vision on a particular point resulting in bumping into things and being 'clumsy', not being able to 'see' objects clearly visible to others and having visuospatial difficulties (e.g. not being able to read text because the letters seem to keep moving). While these difficulties may appear to be related to being able to see, they are in fact a problem with the brain interpreting what it sees correctly. As the condition progresses and more symptoms emerge, it will become apparent to a clinician which type of pathology is causing the problem, and the subtype of dementia becomes clearer. Symptom management can be tailored on this basis.

Rob describes very clearly how Jayne struggled following her accident and, as time moved on, how her cognitive difficulties became more noticeable and diverse. Rob additionally describes how Jayne would 'deny' that she had difficulties. As explained by Dr Hussey, in neurodegenerative conditions it is not uncommon for the person at some point to have no awareness at all of their reduced abilities, their difficulties and their impact on others. This is 'anosognosia' which is a core feature of many dementias. The person will have no awareness that there is something wrong. This is very frustrating for all involved and can impact on a relationship where one party thinks the other is over-reacting and the other thinks the person is under-reacting to a situation or ignoring it completely.

The Admiral Nurse role

The role of the Admiral Nurse is to support people with dementia and their families in dealing with and adjusting to the life changes that come with dementia. Families most often report that they didn't find anyone who knew or understood the story they were telling. Admiral Nurses are specialists in these conditions, of which there are many, and rare diseases in younger people, and will have heard this kind of story many times before. They can help with providing emotional support, practical advice and ongoing monitoring throughout the course of the illness, including prior to diagnosis when support is greatly needed, as Rob's account demonstrates. An Admiral Nurse can work alongside the patient and family to help them come to terms with a diagnosis of dementia and offer guidance and expert advice on symptom management and how to cope. Their role is for the whole family, an often-overlooked aspect of care. The ability of the person with dementia to function well is entirely dependent upon those around them and the support and practical help they provide. It seems essential therefore that Admiral Nurse support for family members, sometimes including young children, parents and siblings, is accessed to help guide the dementia pathway and help coordinate care.

In the case of a rare dementia, a diagnosis may have genetic implications for other family members – very hard to come to terms with or address, particularly when parents may be asking if they contributed to the disease genetically. Siblings may ask how much they are at risk themselves. The ripples of distress are widespread. An Admiral Nurse will be familiar with the questions a family affected by dementia will want to ask and, using their specialist knowledge and experience, together with the shared experience of others in the same situation, can work with the person and family to offer expert advice, understanding, guidance, support and time to listen, advocate and respond. Evidence-based care and advice can act as something of a beacon in stormy times. The Admiral Nursing service recognises this and aims to advise and help from a position of empathy, knowledge, evidence and skill.

REFERENCES

Alzheimer's Society (2014) *Dementia UK Update*. Accessed on 4/5/2022 at www.alzheimers.org.uk/sites/default/files/migrate/downloads/dementia_uk_update.pdf.

Bakker, C., de Vugt, M.E., Vernooij-Dassen, M., van Vliet, D. *et al.* (2010) 'Needs in early onset dementia: A qualitative case from the NeedYD study.' *American Journal of Alzheimer's Disease and Other Dementias 25*, 8, 634–640. doi:10.1177/1533317510385811.

Carter, J.E., Oyebode, J.R. and Koopmans, R.T.C.M. (2018) 'Young-onset dementia and the need for specialist care: A national and international perspective.' *Aging and Mental Health 22*, 4, 468–473. doi:10.1080/13607863.2016.1257563.

Draper, B., Cations, M., White, F., Trollor, J. *et al.* (2016) 'Time to diagnosis in young-onset dementia and its determinants: The INSPIRED study.' *International Journal of Geriatric Psychiatry 31*, 11, 1217–1224. doi:10.1002/gps.4430.

Stamou, V., La Fontaine, J., Gage, H., Jones, B. *et al.* (2019) 'Services for people with young onset dementia: The "Angela" project national UK survey of service use and satisfaction.' *International Journal of Geriatric Medicine 36*, 3, 411–422. doi:10.1002/gps.5437.

RESOURCES AND FURTHER READING
Rare Dementia Support
Specialist support services for people affected by a rare dementia diagnosis. They are based at University College London and provide educational and support meetings tailored to specific conditions, newsletters and telephone or online advice.

www.raredementiasupport.org

Dementia UK
ABOUT YOUNG-ONSET DEMENTIA

www.dementiauk.org/about-dementia/young-onset-dementia/about-young-onset-dementia

CHAPTER 4

'Maintaining independence and autonomy'

BALANCING THE RISKS

WENDY AND SARAH MITCHELL

Wendy

I was diagnosed with dementia on 31 July 2014. I may not have much of a short-term memory any more, but that's one date I never forget as it changed my life. At the time, I was living happily alone in York and in full-time work in the NHS. Naively, I thought services would kick in to help and advise me both financially and emotionally. I had a mortgage, I lived alone, yet there was no help out there. I didn't know the challenges that lay ahead with regard to housing.

After sinking into depression at feeling abandoned by the non-existent services, I began to realise that the only person who was going to help me and my daughters was me. I was forced into early retirement and in a catch-22 situation. I had to sell my house and move to a cheaper area where I could buy a house outright as no one was going to give me a mortgage or allow me to keep my current one. I was forced to move from what I thought was my forever home in York to a quieter village in East Yorkshire

Dementia isn't just about memory – so many of our other senses can be affected as well. One of the first to be affected was my hearing. Loud noises physically hurt my ears. Audiologists are now starting to realise that many people with dementia have hyperacusis, something in common with children with autism. It simply means a sensitivity to certain tones of noise. But they can do something about it by fitting us with ear guards which filter out that specific tone. I was on the waiting list for two years but finally got my magic hearing aids, and they've transformed my life when I'm out and about. So, my quiet village was the ideal solution.

My daughters and I didn't realise at the time that I wasn't capable of choosing an appropriate house. I'd always relished moving in the past and taken on projects and done all the work myself. Suddenly, I chose a house because of the big picture window that overlooked an old paddock, ignoring the two gardens to maintain, the steps up to the front door and at the back of the house, the three bedrooms I didn't need. But we are where we are now, and I adapt it as dementia throws challenges at me.

When I moved, I hadn't appreciated how hard it would be to get used to a new house and learning where I lived. I live in a row of four identical houses, so I had to find a way to make mine different from the others. So, I put two forget-me-not tiles, one each side of my door, and now I know exactly which is mine. I appreciate how people get confused and anxious when they move to a care home – nothing familiar anymore, layouts strange and things not as they were.

I have a tiny kitchen that had two doors which used to confuse the hell out of me as I couldn't remember where the doors led to, so I would spend ages walking round in circles – my solution was simply to take off the doors – I can now see exactly where each exit leads without getting confused. Doors are often a problem for people with dementia. Some prefer them closed to feel safe while others prefer them open. Everyone's different.

I don't see the kitchen cupboards or wardrobes in my bedroom – they just blend into the walls, so I forget there's stuff behind the doors. When I first moved in, my daughters would ask me why I was wearing the same clothes each day, and I said I thought I couldn't have unpacked all my clothes as I couldn't find them, but it was because I couldn't see the wardrobe doors so forgot they were there. Some said I should have bought see-through cupboards – not only are these expensive, but they also look chaotic if you don't keep them mega tidy. So, my solution was to take a photograph of the contents of the cupboards and wardrobes and stick them on the doors. The photos attract my attention and remind me that they have things inside.

Technology now plays a huge part in my life now, enabling me to remain independent. I had never used technology pre-dementia. My newfound friend is 'Alexa'. She puts the lights on upstairs before I climb the stairs to bed. I used to fall frequently in the dark. 'Alexa' reminds me to do certain things at certain times and can calm me down on a bad day by playing me music and reassuringly telling me what day of the week it is... She can even switch the kettle on for me.

It's an advantage that I live alone. Sounds bizarre, I know, but living on my own means that there's no one there to move things around. Because if someone else moves something, to me, it no longer exists or it becomes confusing if I find it in a different place. So, consistency and routine are very important for me. More importantly, it also means I have to find a way to continue to live alone, although I know my daughters are only a WhatsApp away...

Sarah

I hear some sons/daughters talk of their experience and it seems as though the roles have completely reversed: they have become the parent. Yet I don't feel that way. I've certainly had to become more responsible and available for Mum, but that's to help her live independently, not dependently. I have offered to move in before, but I'm glad she declined. I would have made her more dependent by doing things for her.

I've had to stop worrying about her. A couple of years ago, we had the opportunity to go to Italy for four days. We spoke at a dementia conference and then got to spend some time sightseeing. Our lovely guide Molly took us for a short walk along a rocky path to a stunning viewpoint. Mum's gait has been affected by her dementia, and she is at a higher risk of falling than most. At one point, Mum tripped slightly but caught herself and carried on. Molly commented on how relaxed I looked and that I wasn't rushing to grab Mum at any sudden movement. To do this, I have to let go of fear of what could happen. I used to worry constantly about what will happen if she breaks a bone, hits her head or worse. At the end of the day, if I was standing by her side all the time, wrapping her in bubble wrap, she would not have any joy in that walk. So, I let it happen. Whatever is going to happen will happen. As long as there is joy, it is worth doing. I must admit, I sometimes walk in front so I can't see the little stumbles...

I am writing from the perspective of a daughter who has always had a fiercely independent mother. Everyone's relationships are different. Your loved one may have always depended on you for certain things. If this is the case, I'm not suggesting you change the way you have always done things. However, perhaps just keep this question in mind: would I always have done this, or am I changing my behaviour due to their dementia? For anyone who may be at the beginning of this journey, I would suggest stepping back and not jumping in to help. It took a lot of soul searching for me to mentally, as well as physically, do that. It did not come naturally. When you love someone and you know you can do something, you just want to do it! But, actually, the most loving thing you can do is help them keep their sense of self by letting them be.

SPECIALIST COMMENTARY

Professor Julian C. Hughes, Honorary Professor, Bristol Medical School, Bristol Population Health Science Institute, University of Bristol, UK and Visiting Professor, Policy, Ethics and Life Sciences (PEALS) Research Centre, Newcastle University, UK

Is autonomy what we want?

There are problems with the notion of respect for autonomy. We might wish to start by acknowledging that autonomy is sometimes seen as the key principle in ethics. In the world of medical ethics, which it might be better to call clinical ethics (to signify that ethical issues do not occur only for doctors), people talk about the four principles (Beauchamp and Childress 2013). They are useful principles, too, when it comes to day-to-day ethical decisions of the sort that Wendy and Sarah have faced. The principles are: respect for autonomy, beneficence (doing good), non-maleficence (avoiding harm) and justice (being fair). But it is often felt that respect for autonomy should trump the other principles. This is because, at least in liberal democratic societies, the person's right to be in charge of her or his own destiny seems paramount. 'Autonomy', after all, means 'self-rule'.

Wendy and Sarah's account has already shown how respecting

autonomy and beneficence or non-maleficence can clash as principles. Wendy is inclined to walk without support. Of course, Sarah is concerned that she should do good to her mother and avoid harm. Both of these inclinations would make her wish to support her mother walking over rocky terrain. But, if not asked, to do so would not respect Wendy's ability to make her own mind up, to show autonomy. Sarah makes the decision, therefore, that her mother's autonomy should be respected. She does not wish to infantilise her mother. Of course, if Wendy were her young child, Sarah might well take the decision to hold her hand even if she objected; even so, at some point the autonomy of the youngster must also be respected, and (as Sarah suggests in connection with older people) different parents might take different decisions about when this should occur. Respect for a person's autonomy is part of what it is to respect dignity, independence, freedom, equality and, quite generally, his or her rights as a human being.

I hope this all sounds fine and dandy. But actually it's not! Or not completely. I've already said there are (at least) two things that might seem dodgy. The first was this: the person's right to be in charge of her or his own destiny seems paramount; and the second was my talk of respect for autonomy being part of what it is to respect a person's rights quite generally. I still want to say that respect for autonomy is very important. Wendy is a good example of this. She would not wish for her daughters to barge in and take control of all aspects of her life, and nor would they wish to. Life would become too circumspect for Wendy. There would be no room for the sort of feeling of flourishing that we all enjoy when we have coped with things ourselves and made our own decisions.

Nevertheless, it is not completely clear that the right to be in charge of your own destiny should always be paramount. What if a person starts to do things they wish to do but that endanger other people? What if someone living with a diagnosis of dementia loves walking but starts to get lost? As Wendy has discovered, she can maintain her independence by using technology, and we should respect her autonomous decisions to do so. A person who gets lost might also use technology to lessen the chances of harm. But what if that person starts walking across roads without looking? At some point, the safety and wellbeing of others will start to gain paramountcy.

What about my talk of the person's rights quite generally? Well, we also have rights around our dignity. If I become incontinent, for instance, for a while it might be up to me when I get changed. But at some point my dignity might require that others force the issue. My inclination might be not to get changed. But while respecting this inclination is indeed *part of* my right to respect as a human being, it's not the whole story. I also have a right to be kept clean and safe from infections, and respecting my dignity might entail sometimes forcing the issue of care and overriding my autonomy.

The point is that autonomy is not the only pebble on the beach. More than that, we rarely ever have complete autonomy. I might think I have autonomy to sit here and type on my computer. But this requires electricity. I've also required food and drink during the day. The banana I had for lunch was certainly not grown in my garden! The truth is, none of us is completely autonomous. Indeed, we are dependent. We can go so far as to say that in order to exercise our autonomy, we often have to accept our dependency (on the people, for instance, who provide the electricity and who grow and ship the bananas). In an excellent book on this subject, George Agich (2003) suggested that autonomy and dependency might almost be regarded as different sides of the same coin. My autonomy often depends on other things or other people; contrariwise, in the best of worlds, my dependency still allows room for respect of my autonomy.

One way around this has been to talk instead of 'relational' autonomy (Mackenzie and Stoljar 2000). This acknowledges that our autonomous decisions typically involve relationships with others. Either they depend on or they affect other people. Wendy's decisions – for example, about where she lives – affect the lives of her daughters. Sarah's decision to hang back and not to intervene in her mother's life affects Wendy and potentially (e.g. if she were to have a fall and fracture something) others in the family. Interventions by health and social care professionals also affect the whole family (as do a lack of interventions, which Wendy has sadly experienced). The point is that our autonomous decisions are made in the context of relationships. Therefore, the notion of relational autonomy makes a lot of sense.

One worry about this is that 'relational' autonomy is simply not real autonomy. Some might say that it's just an excuse for others to get involved. It could be suggested or thought that Wendy cannot make a decision unless it involves Sarah. Relational autonomy inevitably brings in the family; but since we are 'in relationship' with numerous others, it might mean that all and sundry get involved in our decisions. Respect for Wendy's *relational* autonomy might mean that what Wendy actually wants is simply ignored in favour of what everyone else wants. We need to stipulate that Wendy remains centre stage. But it is then difficult to do justice to the fact that Wendy, like all of us, is dependent on others. Dementia makes this truth starker.

So what is to be done? Well, I think we have to see ourselves as real people – or, better still, as real persons. Personhood suggests the ethical and legal standing that real people have *just because* they are human beings. I have characterised personhood in terms of situated embodied agency (Hughes 2011). In brief, to be a person is to be situated in numerous fields, bringing in our personal histories, our family and social backgrounds, the legal systems we live in, the geography and economic realities that affect us, our moral and religious beliefs and so on. We are also bodies, with different potentials, but subject to illness with which we cope on the basis of the resources (physical, psychological, social and spiritual) available to us (i.e. reflecting our situatedness). Our agency refers to our ability to do things, albeit this is enhanced or curtailed by – it is more or less autonomous depending on – our situated embodiment.

If this all sounds a little theoretical, it should be noted that it perfectly describes the situation facing Wendy and Sarah. Wendy's narrative (in which she is situated) is one of independence. As an agent, she makes her own decisions, but she has the support of her family. It is in the context of her caring daughters that she lives. They are concerned but respect the degree to which she wishes to exercise her autonomous agency. Of course, Sarah and her sister(s) are also situated and have their own narratives, values, anxieties and the like, which inevitably interact with the situatedness of Wendy. Her increasing dependency is recognised by Wendy herself (she knows how much she depends on 'Alexa', as well as on the tricks she has learned to help her remember what might be in her cupboards and wardrobes). The state of her body – whether to do with her hearing, vision or tendency to fall – is also recognised. At every point, and especially if decisions are required, the whole of the surrounding context comes into play. This doesn't mean that others take over from Wendy – far from it.

But the complexity of the decisions and the risks that become apparent are recognised and faced up to both by Wendy and by Sarah. Furthermore, it is not being suggested that the compromises which Wendy and Sarah have negotiated (not necessarily overtly, but covertly) should be regarded as binding for others. We are all situated – bodily, psychologically, socially and spiritually – in different ways. We all have different values. The paths we navigate, the risks we take and the ways we respect autonomy are all differently embedded and require skill and nuance to negotiate in the real-life situations we face.

ADMIRAL NURSE ADVICE

Lucy Chamberlain, Admiral Nurse, Royal British Legion

Everyday life holds many potential hazards for all of us that we are subconsciously risk-assessing all the time – crossing the road, using kitchen gadgets and so on. We are constantly taking these small risks because we know we can manage them, and they give us a broader quality of life. Usually, we assume that the people around us can manage those risks too, but if dementia is added into the mix, it can feel tricky to get the balance right between enabling people to remain independent and taking those universal risks on the one hand and the feeling that they need protecting from harm on the other.

Prior to receiving the diagnosis, most people with dementia will have been living full and independent lives, and no one around them may have been worried about any 'risks'. This might mean that sometimes we don't notice when skills are changing or diminishing, and then a crisis can occur, such as being a victim of a financial scam, accidents and injuries, all of which can be heart-breaking for family carers with the notion that these things could potentially have been avoided. However, taking over decision making and trying to remove any possible risks can lead to the person with dementia feeling resentful, reducing their quality of life and becoming deskilled and deteriorating more quickly (Rapaport et al. 2020).

So how do we strike a balance? 'Positive risk taking' is the approach that allows us to weigh up the perceived risks of harm to the person (of doing something) against the perceived risks to them of the negative impact on their quality of life, independence and rights (in not doing something). This means we need to consider collaboratively with the person with dementia, families, friends, perhaps even neighbours and locally involved services to work out what any potential problems might be, and how we can work together to overcome them (Morgan and Andrews 2016). It is well worth setting up a Property and Financial Affairs Lasting Power of Attorney (LPA) with trusted people and discussing finances as early as possible, as well as a Health and Welfare LPA where everyone gets a chance to explore the person's wishes and feelings, so that the person with dementia can be reassured that these will be followed (see Chapter 5).

There are a lot of technological developments that have made life much easier for all of us and which can be easily adapted. For example, a person with dementia can continue to safely manage their debit card and money, but with the safeguard of a nominated person (perhaps an adult child) who can be added to the account to keep an eye on banking activity and activate an alert if they feel something is wrong.

There are many gadgets now that can be used to mitigate the risks where a person with dementia lives alone. Devices can be used that monitor certain aspects of the home, such as sensors that can detect and then stop overflowing taps or turn off the gas supply if a burner is left unlit. There are alarms for doors that can notify someone if they are opened, trackers that can help find people when they are lost, wearable falls detectors, automated medicines systems, sensor lights and even CCTV in the house that can be accessed by smartphone. All of these can enable a person with dementia to live as independently as possible and remain safe. More low-tech ideas include the use of photos – as we saw in Wendy's case – or signs and notices on cupboards, doors and wardrobes; calendars; memory clocks; memo boards; notices and reminder alarms.

Knowing when to implement these aids and adaptations is the key to person-centred care. For some people with dementia, the use of these methods may feel too intrusive, especially if they are not at the centre of the discussions on their possible use or if put in place too soon. For others, they can be a good way for the person with dementia to carry on living independently, while reassuring family members that there will be a way to be notified if help is needed in their absence. Regularly reviewing and talking through the plans made together will help to adapt and update the use of such aids as required. The usefulness of some of these aids will change over time, so it is important to review periodically.

REFERENCES

Agich, G.J. (2003) *Dependence and Autonomy in Old Age: An Ethical Framework for Long-Term Care*. Cambridge: Cambridge University Press.

Beauchamp, T.L. and Childress, J.F. (2013) *Principles of Biomedical Ethics* (7th edition). Oxford and New York: Oxford University Press.

Hughes, J.C. (2011) *Thinking through Dementia*. Oxford: Oxford University Press.

Mackenzie, C. and Stoljar, N. (eds) (2000) *Relational Autonomy: Feminist Essays on Autonomy, Agency and the Social Self*. New York: Oxford University Press.

Morgan, S. and Andrews, N. (2016) 'Positive risk-taking: From rhetoric to reality.' *The Journal of Mental Health Training, Education and Practice 11*, 2, 122–132. doi:10.1108/JMHTEP-09-2015-0045.

Rapaport, P., Burton, A., Leverton, M. *et al.* (2020) '"I just keep thinking that I don't want to rely on people." A qualitative study of how people living with dementia achieve and maintain independence at home: Stakeholder perspectives.' *BMC Geriatrics 20*, 5. doi:10.1186/s12877-019-1406-6.

RESOURCES AND FURTHER READING
Assistive technology

Most gadgets can be found by searching online for 'dementia assistive technology'. However, it is often useful if there is the opportunity to discuss these aids with those that are knowledgeable about their practical utility and implementation or their cost. Many social services departments can advise on what assistive technologies are available to you in your area or who you can go to.

Alzheimer's Society
WHAT IS ASSISTIVE TECHNOLOGY?

www.alzheimers.org.uk/get-support/staying-independent/what-assistive-technology

ALZHEIMER'S SOCIETY'S VIEW ON ASSISTIVE TECHNOLOGY

www.alzheimers.org.uk/about-us/policy-and-influencing/what-we-think/assistive-technology

CHAPTER 5

'Planning ahead is so overwhelming'

ADVANCE CARE PLANNING

Marion Small (pseudonym)

David and I married after a brief romance. Both our families said it wouldn't last as they said we were too young and did not really know each other well enough. Well, here we are, having recently celebrated our golden wedding anniversary and still going strong. We proved them all wrong. We also went on to have three beautiful children: Amanda, Louise and Clifford. Sadly, Louise died of meningitis when she was 13 years old. This had a devastating effect on us all, and we still miss her dreadfully – but life goes on, so they say. If I can say this, after such a devastating loss, we have been fortunate in that we have both had our health and were looking forward to our retirement, both of us having been in teaching for most of our working lives. However, sadly, David started to have problems with his memory about two years into his much-anticipated retirement. As a teacher of mathematics, he was obviously highly numerate and managed our joint accounts, pension funds and stuff very well initially. I had always left the management of the family finances to him; I always used to say, 'No point us both putting effort into the same things!' Strangely, he started to forget various payments (not like him as he always hated to think he owed money to anybody) or on occasions he would even try to pay again.

We were both aware that something was very wrong and went jointly to see our family doctor. We both had the same GP for years. Hearing stories now, we must have been one of the fortunate ones in a way as the doctor recognised that David's behaviour was not normal for him and very quickly referred him for a memory assessment. After three months of tests and appointments, David was diagnosed with a mixed dementia of Alzheimer's disease and vascular dementia by the psychiatrist of the memory clinic at our local hospital. The psychiatrist said that they were discharging him as they had completed their tests and given him his diagnosis. One of the final things she said was that we should think about planning ahead for David's future care and gave us a brief leaflet about Lasting Power of Attorney; confusingly, there seemed to be two types, so which one should we have?

Ed, a friend of ours, whose wife also has dementia, told us about how they were being helped to develop an advance care plan to identify the future care wishes of his wife. We were not sure if this was the same as a Lasting Power of Attorney, though – surely the psychiatrist would have told us? Ed seems to have a professional who meets with him and his wife to help them with this. Is this a service that is available for everyone with a diagnosis of dementia? I don't seem to be getting anywhere with this. David and I are very confused about what all this means and how to go about this planning ahead, but we want to make sure we have thought of everything going forward as we do not want to have to rely on the children; they have their own lives. It is all so overwhelming.

SPECIALIST COMMENTARY

Karen Harrison Dening, Head of Research and Publications, Dementia UK, and Professor of Dementia Nursing, De Montfort University, Leicester

What is advance care planning and why is it important for people with dementia?

Advance care planning (ACP) has been in existence for a long time, although its use is more common in other life-limiting diseases, such as cancer. It is a process of communication and preparation for or deciding about your future care and treatment, and may or may not include its documentation. An ACP is planned for a time when the person has the capacity to consider their wishes and preferences and to make decisions about care and treatment in advance of a time where they may not have the capacity to do so. The potential benefits of ACP include higher-quality end-of-life care, a greater compliance with a person's end-of-life wishes, as well as a reduction in the stress, anxiety and depression in family members that survive them.

Developing an ACP usually involves people who are important to the person with dementia, such as family members, friends and their health and/or social care team at the time. Ideally, ACP discussions are not a one-off conversation or process but several developing and repeated conversations about future wishes and preferences. An ACP provides people with dementia the opportunity to talk about their values, to reflect upon many things, even the meanings and consequences of potential or future serious illness scenarios added to their dementia, such as pneumonia or stroke.

Capacity to make decisions about care

Thinking about the future is something that we often give little consideration to, especially as we go about our busy lives. A diagnosis such as dementia often makes people pause and consider the impact this may have on their future. People with dementia and their families, as with anyone else diagnosed with a life-limiting condition, may wish to make sure that everything is in order from the point of receiving the diagnosis. Others may need time and support to adjust, but want to have information about who they can contact to discuss any questions or concerns when they are ready to do so.

Knowing what a person's wishes and preferences are, when they no longer have capacity or are able to express them, provides clear guidance for health and social care professionals, and reassures families, when faced with having to make potentially difficult decisions on behalf of the person with dementia, that they can be confident these decisions lead to care and treatment in line with what the person's wishes and preferences would have been.

When to start an advance care plan

People with dementia should be offered and supported to have advance care planning conversations as soon as possible after their diagnosis, or in the earlier stages of the illness. However, many health-care professionals might find conversations about end-of-life care and advance care planning difficult to hold. It is too easy to give an information leaflet or to 'signpost' to another service when you do not have the experience or confidence to start this process off – this may have been what happened in the case of David's psychiatrist.

An ACP does not have to be a written document, although this is the surest way of ensuring the person's wishes and preferences are more widely known; however, simply having an open and honest discussion about they do or don't want for care in the future is still of value.

Let's consider some of the terms used

There are many terms used that can be confusing for people with dementia and their families in terms of what each offers. Advance care planning is generally considered to comprise of three main elements:

- statements about future needs and wishes

- advance decision to refuse treatment (ADRT)

- Lasting Power of Attorney (LPA) – of which there are two types: personal welfare and finances.

As Marion and David were finding, it can initially seem a difficult thing to think and talk about, especially when you are not quite sure what an ACP is, where to start or where to get help. Most people may already have thought about some of the things that an ACP might embrace and may have even talked about them with their family, friends and caregivers.

Advance statements about future needs and wishes

An advance statement explains your wishes, views and preferences for the future. An advance statement might include where you wish to live and be cared for as you near the end of your life, or the type of care and support you wish to receive. One could also include other things, such as who you would wish to care for a pet or social activities you would wish to continue (see the Admiral Nurse section below for more).

If you decide to write down your advance statement, decide the best place to keep it so that people can access it when needed – for example, your GP, relatives or friends. Where possible, these wishes should be complied with; there would need to be good reasons if they are not. If there are reasons why a person's wishes and preferences cannot be met, then a best interests decision should made to record why not. As part of the law (Mental Capacity Act), the healthcare professional in charge of the care of the person with dementia or an appointed person must make decisions about your treatment and care based on what they believe is in your best interests.

Often people may tell others that they want to stay in their home and not move to a care home, but it may not always be possible to follow this. For example, it may no longer be in a person's best interests to stay in their home for a variety of reasons, such as their family carer is no longer able to care for them at home, even with support. It is better if wishes and preferences are discussed widely from the outset so that when facing potentially difficult situations, such as when a move to a care home is the most appropriate care setting, a best interest decision may be made taking into consideration the person's wishes while recognising the current context.

Advance decision to refuse treatment

An ADRT ensures that in a given situation (previously described and documented), the person is not forced to receive treatment that they did not want. If the document is correctly worded, you can refuse treatments, *but* in law you cannot *request* treatments. Treatment that can be refused include life-sustaining treatment, even if in so refusing, it will hasten death – for example, refusing cardiac resuscitation in certain circumstances.

ADRTs are legally binding as long as they meet certain conditions, such as what treatments and in what circumstances (see the 'Resources and further reading' section at the end of this chapter for more guidance) to make it valid. When properly written, doctors are required to follow it and the ADRT will only come into force when the person is no longer able to make decisions for themselves and at a time when needed.

Lasting Power of Attorney

Lasting Power of Attorney (LPA) is a legal document that gives another adult the authority to make certain decisions on a person's behalf, if they become unable to do so for themselves. There are two types of LPA: one for property and finances and the other for health and welfare. Each type of LPA has its own form, which can be filled in online or in hard copy (see the 'Resources and further reading' section at the end of this chapter). Whichever way you choose, the form needs to be printed, signed and registered with the Office of the Public Guardian to become valid. As with an ACP and ADRT, LPAs can only be developed when the person has the capacity to do so.

An Enduring Power of Attorney (made before the change to LPA), if correctly filled in, is still valid if appropriately registered. However, an Enduring Power of Attorney only covered property and financial decisions and did not include health and welfare. Marion and David don't necessarily need to seek legal advice, or use a solicitor, in order to make an LPA; many people complete the form themselves as the forms come with comprehensive guidance.

Changes can be made along the way to all of these documents while the person has capacity to make any changes but become active when the person loses capacity.

Who can help us to plan ahead?

The immediate post-diagnostic period is a very important time for families affected by dementia in being supported to face their life with the diagnosis and what that might mean, such as prognosis and potential future needs. These can be difficult conversations for some families and professionals to have, and it is important to balance these difficult conversations with a hopeful attitude of realistic optimism that the disease can be managed.

Researchers have emphasised the need for a single healthcare provider to take on a central role in facilitating ACP for families affected by dementia. This is also recommended in UK policy and guidance (National Institute for Health and Care Excellence (NICE) 2018). There are professionals in many areas that can support a person with the diagnosis of dementia and their families to commence ACP, such as Admiral Nurses (specialist dementia nurses). The service that made the diagnosis – for example, a memory clinic, neurology clinic or your GP – may be able to provide information on what local services are available.

ADMIRAL NURSE ADVICE

Angela Moore, Consultant Admiral Nurse, Dementia UK, and **Maggie Fay**, Admiral Nurse, Rutland County Council

When diagnosed with a progressive, life-limiting condition such as dementia, you may have contact with many health and social care professionals who can offer you information and advice about thinking and planning for your future care. Although in this chapter we are discussing advance care planning in relation to dementia care, it is important to recognise that we can all develop our own advance care plan.

It is quite normal to feel overwhelmed and reluctant to question the support or advice you are offered, as we see in Marion and David's story. Also, as a family carer, Marion's thoughts and feelings about considering advance planning may be different to David's or those of other family members. A person's views on future care decisions (goals of care) may also vary depending on other things, such as previous life experiences, experiences of death of other family members over the years, spiritual beliefs, etc. For some people, these conversations may be less comfortable to have than for others. Often discussions may be easier to hold if helped or facilitated by a professional, who can explain terminology using the right words and choose the right time and setting in which to start the conversation. In Marion's case, it may be a good place to start in thinking about her own wishes and preferences, what care and treatment would she like or not, and who she would want to speak for her if she was unable to do so in the future. Many couples may have had various conversations throughout their relationship about the future if they become ill, but perhaps they have not really taken note. They may have seen a drama on TV where a character experiences a health condition or a painful death, and they may have said, 'I don't want that to happen to me', for example.

When is the best time to think about ACP?

Thinking about when to start advance care planning will be different for everyone. Many people will have already thought about their future wishes and preferences as part of completing a will or in funeral planning. However, these are largely making decisions in advance of your death about what you want to happen to your possessions after you die or to your body after death. An advance care plan is more about what you want to happen to you while still alive but unable to make your own decisions. It is not unusual for people to only consider ACP when they are faced with a health crisis. They may find themselves being asked by health professionals to make decisions about their care now or in the future, but this can be difficult for a person with dementia, especially if they have lost capacity to do so, or for a family member who may not be sure what the person may or may not have wanted. Talking about ACP should ideally be commenced while the person with dementia has capacity to share their thoughts and wishes.

Who should make the advance care plan – person with dementia, family carer or both?

Ideally, the person with dementia should be supported to consider their future wishes and preferences as early after the diagnosis as possible. However, most people with dementia make their plans in partnership with those close to them and supported by any healthcare professional they are in contact with. This may be (for example) an Admiral Nurse, GP or social worker. If the person with dementia prefers others to take the lead, this is fine and not unusual. In Marion's case, she might consider other family members who may be able to offer her support; she may have a close relationship with her eldest child, Amanda. Amanda may feel more confident and able to support or initiate such a conversation with her father and so enable Marion to develop confidence to engage or lead in future conversations. Often when such discussions are held with several family members together, there may emerge a sense of clarity and increasing awareness of what the person with dementia wishes for.

How do I get started?

David seems to be willing to have a conversation about his care in the future, but it may be a new and strange thing for some to think about, so it is important to give them every opportunity to do so. Consider the time of day you initiate the conversation; choose a time when the person with dementia is at their best, most alert and less likely to be distressed. Choose an environment that is comfortable, familiar and free from distractions. For many, the most comfortable place is home; ACP conversations do not require a clinical setting. Always make sure that the person has the best possible chance for good communication, whether that is the person with dementia or another family member, so ensure that the person is comfortable and undistracted (not in pain, cold, hungry, etc.), and if they wear a hearing aid, ensure it is working well.

How you position yourself is important, too. Ensure you have good eye contact; this will enable you to observe for any non-verbal signs of discomfort or distress, such as changes to facial expressions and body language. These may be indicators that you need to stop and move on to something very different. Talk in a tone that is audible to the person so they can hear you, and don't rush the conversation. You can hold such discussions over several days or weeks so as not to tire them. It is always good to check that you have understood their wishes, and a good way of doing this is to repeat back to them by slightly rephrasing, possibly saying, 'So, what I think you are telling me is that...' This will also help them to review what they are saying when they hear what is said back to them.

The language used can affect the response of the person with dementia, so avoid unnecessary jargon or health terminology and use terms that the person is familiar with – even the term 'advance care planning' might need an initial explanation. Although ACP is not just about dying, you might want to consider how the person previously described death and dying. This is quite important as words such as 'pass away' or 'passing on' may not be terms or expressions you use but they may be those the person with dementia has used in the past.

Thinking about spiritual needs

When planning for the future, some people wish to think about their spiritual needs. These will be different for everyone and may or may not be associated solely with religion. This presents an opportunity to discuss the person's individual values and beliefs, what is important to them, and enable them to explore their future hopes and fears. An opportunity to talk about their spiritual and/or religious needs may provide them with reassurance or a sense of wellbeing and peace.

Does it have to be a written document?

Writing down the ACP can provide really useful information to others involved in the care of the person with dementia, both now and in the future, such as family members or the health and social care team. An ACP may enable them to provide better support as they will have a good understanding of future wishes and goals of care. The ACP could be a written document or in a digital format that is kept on the person's healthcare records. Either way, it is important that it is shared with all involved in the care of the person with dementia so it can also be followed in times of emergency.

What if the person with dementia doesn't want to talk about it?

It is OK not to want to talk about future care wishes; advance care planning is not mandatory. It may be frightening or difficult for some people to think about the end of life, and thinking ahead can be difficult for some. Marion and David may have stated in passing conversations things that they wouldn't want to happen to them or something they would want to happen. Sometimes such instances can be used to initiate or broaden a conversation. Remember that advance care planning is often a gradual process that evolves over time.

What things can I include in an advance care plan?

There is no right way and no real beginning or end, but taking that first step can sometimes seem like a hurdle to get over. There are many guides and templates that you can use when starting to think about what to include in an ACP. A person's long held beliefs and values are often a good starting point; thinking about what matters most to them while also using one of the resources detailed below can help kickstart the process. Things to consider might be:

- In the light of a diagnosis of dementia, what matters to you (person with dementia and/or family carer)? What are your fears, your wishes, your goals of care? What would be a good death for you?

- Consider previous life experiences and the deaths of other family members. Did these have meaning for how you see your own future health and care wishes?

- Talking about death, dying and bereavement can be hard for some people. It can feel awkward or uncomfortable, and sometimes you just don't know what to say. Challenging the taboo of death and dying is at the heart of the Dying Matters campaign (see the 'Resources and further reading' section at the end of this chapter).

- Think about what treatments and care you may or may not wish to receive if you become ill in the future, such as if you develop cancer, have a heart attack or a stroke.

- Where does the person with dementia wish to be cared for? Where would they prefer to die?

- How well do you understand the condition of dementia? Think about what you already know and what you would like to know. You may need to ask questions of your health and social care team, GP or Admiral Nurse about what you might expect as the dementia progresses and how you might plan ahead.

- When thinking about death and dying, we often worry about those left behind. What would you want for them?

- Ask for support from professionals who are skilled in supporting ACP conversations at any point.

- Above all, be kind to yourself and take your time to plan.

In summary

Advance care planning helps us to think ahead and have a sense of control over the care we would or would not like to receive should we become ill and not be able to express this at the time. An ACP can also provide information that helps those around the person with dementia to support them in accordance with their wishes and preferences as they near the end of their lives. Advance care planning can support the person to live well and die well in their preferred place of death, and ensure care is consistent with their values, goals and preferences. However, it is important to recognise that sometimes a person with dementia may wish to make decisions that a carer feels are unwise; this does not mean they are wrong. It is important for the family carer to also think about who can support them to manage their own feelings during this process.

REFERENCES

National Institute for Health and Care Excellence (NICE) (2018) 'Dementia: assessment, management and support for people living with dementia and their carers.' NICE guideline [NG97]. Accessed on 5/5/2022 at www.nice.org.uk/guidance/ng97.

RESOURCES AND FURTHER READING
NHS Guidance
MY FUTURE WISHES: ADVANCE CARE PLANNING (ACP) FOR PEOPLE WITH DEMENTIA IN ALL CARE SETTINGS

www.england.nhs.uk/publication/my-future-wishes-advance-care-planning-acp-for-people-with-dementia-in-all-care-settings

Dying Matters
The Dying Matters campaign is working to create an open culture in which we're comfortable talking about death, dying and bereavement.

www.hospiceuk.org/our-campaigns/dying-matters

Dementia UK
A GUIDE TO ADVANCE CARE PLANNING AND A TEMPLATE FROM WHICH YOU CAN DEVELOP YOUR OWN ADVANCE CARE PLAN

www.dementiauk.org/get-support/legal-and-financial-information/advance-care-planning

Advance Decisions to Refuse Treatment

www.nhs.uk/conditions/end-of-life-care/advance-decision-to-refuse-treatment

Lasting Power of Attorney
Office of the Public Guardian: A free booklet is available on each type of the Lasting Power of Attorney. Forms and information about Lasting Power of Attorney are available to download.

www.gov.uk/power-of-attorney

CHAPTER 6

'Once he got a diagnosis, the girls had to believe'

DISTANCE AND DENIAL OF DEMENTIA

Gina Hyde (pseudonym)

I first became concerned when my husband and I retired from our jobs. Odd things started to happen. Concern turned to worry about my husband's behaviours, and I tried to confide in my daughters. However, they would always ascribe the changes in their father to other things and put them down to old age, but he was only in his middle years. The changes in my husband were that he became low on empathy, easy to rise to irritability and anger, melodramatic and controlling of me. Our daughters did not live in the family home by this time, so they only had my word on what was happening to their father. They did not seem to believe me.

Three months before he eventually got his diagnosis of behavioural variant frontotemporal dementia (BvFTD), my eldest child said to me, 'Dad is not that bad, Mum.' Once he got a diagnosis, the girls *had* to believe that he was ill, and the odd things that they observed were now explained. But still they did not seem to believe what I was telling them. My husband and I had had years of an inequitable and bickering marriage, yet all of a sudden it was not OK to bicker with him because he was ill, but even more so because he had dementia. It then became 'OK' to blame the dementia and for them to say, 'He looks *fine* to me' if ever I tried to talk to them about it.

The girls acted in a supportive way, saying things like 'I can't even imagine how hard this is', but they seemed to hoard examples of things

I was handling wrong. We had always had the type of relationship where the girls felt free to approach me on all manner of things. However, as time went on, all three started to criticise different aspects of my caregiving. The emphasis shifted from 'supporting Mum' to 'poor Dad'. This was after their father had hit me because I told him not to kick his mum's dogs.

This was devastating to me, especially on top of all the previous criticisms. The girls did not feel that I was trying as hard as I could do to keep their dad at home. They seemed to believe that I might put him into a home before *they* thought it necessary. I eventually did have to place him in a care home, with the effect that the girls' denial of how things had become escalated. To the point that one daughter felt he should be placed in a home central to the family, not one that had experience of managing residents with BvFTD behaviours. His move into the home was followed with many accusatory comments, such as 'You are using your stress as an excuse to throw him in a home', 'You were mean to him', 'You never take our advice' and 'You should have taken antidepressants when all this started if you were having trouble handling our dad'.

There was no belief in me or my motives and judgement, and they showed no understanding of the behaviours I lived with. They showed no trust in me to continue to be responsible, do the right thing and to keep their father at home for as long as I could. I begged for their trust. I told them I had years of being responsible and compassionate, loving and helping their dad – why did they now doubt me? Silence. They made me feel like I was not doing a good job caring for their dad. They didn't understand what I was going through and would just say, 'I can't even imagine.' They did make some suggestions over the years, but I acted on very few since they were unworkable for us. This made them withdraw from me more. They did not appreciate quite what it was like to live with their father, because when they visited, there were always more people to provide the support. They didn't have to cave in to his demands as I had to. They never offered to take him out or for him to visit their homes.

Some time after my husband went into care, the girls made their peace with it and began to behave as though things between us were normal, with all the unpleasantness in the past. We resumed a more normal pre-BvFTD relationship, but it was now superficial, with no mention of problems past. Their lack of compassion and support of me was devastating, and still things are really not what they were.

SPECIALIST COMMENTARY

Dr Rheinhard Guss, Consultant Clinical Psychologist, Clinical Neuropsychologist

Denial as a coping mechanism

Denial as a coping mechanism in the face of overwhelming anxiety was first suggested and described by Sigmund Freud in the late 19th century. It has since been developed mainly in the psychoanalytic field (meaning that the focus is on the unconscious mind rather than the conscious). Our brains are incredible in the way they function, and they have the ability to use automatic filters to support our likes and beliefs, both about ourselves and about the world outside. Anything in contradiction is more likely to be dismissed or ignored. For example, people who smoke know that it is harmful to their health, but because they like the effect of smoking, their brain filters out these negative thoughts. Denial is one of the unconscious 'defence mechanisms' we use to avoid anxiety and emotional pain, and to ensure that we are 'acceptable' to others.

Denial is often seen in people who have dementia themselves. This can lead to conflicts with partners and families due to the insistence that 'everything is fine' and that there 'is no problem', leading to refusal of cooperation with diagnosis or with help and care. However, family carers can also face denial by other family members who may find it equally frightening or traumatic to acknowledge the presence of a dementia in a loved one.

Stigma and dementia

Despite the efforts of many countries' dementia strategies to address the stigma and social exclusion of dementia, the word itself continues to invoke fear in a way only comparable to cancer. It has been found to be the most feared medical condition in the over-50s today (Alzheimer's Society 2016). While cancer has become increasingly treatable and survivable over the past 50 years or so, the same is not the case for dementia. And while there are now many examples of people leading active and fulfilling lives despite a dementia diagnosis, the wider perception of dementia remains that of a 'death sentence', of 'losing their mind', of a 'slow descent into forgetting everything about oneself and one's history'. The dominant imagery is that of the very late stages of dementia, of helplessness and an undignified inability to look after one's most basic needs. This collective image of dementia makes the thought of it particularly frightening and thus a prime candidate for defence mechanisms such as denial to be triggered.

A further factor adding to the perception of dementia as an existential threat that cannot be processed, and therefore has to be denied in order to be able to continue to cope, can often be found in the stories passed on in family history. There is often a relative who had been exposed to the draconian, neglectful or abusive regimes of poor care for older people, people with mental health difficulties or, in particular, with dementia. People with difficulties that could nowadays be easily recognised as symptoms of a developing dementia, who were seen as unable to look after themselves, might have gone to the 'poor house' or the 'back wards' of the local mental hospital, where they eventually died. While health and social care systems, despite their ongoing problems, are today very much improved, the impressions and attitudes that create and guide such fearful imagery are developed very early on in life, and are often not consciously reflected upon, again increasing the likelihood of denial being employed to cope.

Fears of inheriting dementia
Another aspect of dementia that often fuels fears and defence mechanisms in families is the ongoing perception of dementia as a hereditary illness linked to genetics. The percentage of directly inherited cases of dementia is, in reality, minute. Alzheimer's disease, the most frequent form of dementia, is hardly ever inherited; nonetheless, the question about any relatives having had dementia remains in the diagnostic interviews, often adding to the impression that it may be passed on in families. Behavioural variant frontotemporal dementia, as in this case, has a larger proportion of genetic transmission, although this is also more likely at an earlier age. With the notion of the inheritability of dementia, relatives – in particular children or grandchildren – may

be particularly fearful that what they see in their parent or grandparent is what they will in due course experience themselves. The more frightening they find this, the greater the chance that denial will be used to cope with these aversive notions.

Distance of family members

Living some distance away from the person with a dementia diagnosis can add to denial in friends or relatives who see the person infrequently, perhaps for relatively short visits, or speak with them on the phone. Telephone conversations with parents who live a long distance away, as described in Gina's case, often follow a predictable script that the participants have developed over a long period of time. Having a regular pattern of who talks first, the questions that are asked and the topics that are covered can be very helpful for the person with dementia to function at their best, while the other party will not experience any particular changes that they would identify as related to dementia.

While the partner or carer at home will, of course, experience the difficult moments or challenging periods with the person with dementia, relatives who live away will not usually be party to these and have to take the word of the carer for this. People with dementia will often present very well for the duration of a visit from an adult child, a friend or relative. Family carers can find this difficult and feel the person is 'putting on a show' for the occasion, while reserving the difficulties for times when there is no additional help. The tendency to be on our best behaviour during social occasions, to mobilise all our reserves, is not unique to people with dementia and is a universal human mechanism to maintain our social bonds. While rarely employed as a conscious means to deceive visitors about any dementia-related difficulties, it does, however, put family carers in a difficult position, especially when faced with friends or relatives who are denying that there is anything amiss, or who may be looking for comforting and reassuring evidence to alleviate their own anxieties or feelings of guilt.

In Gina's case, another approach to take might be the systemic perspective taken by practitioners of family therapy. We know that the arrival of dementia in families tends to 'force the issues' and bring to the fore the difficulties in family relationships and communication that have always existed in this system. This may be all the more so when faced with frontotemporal dementia (FTD), which tends to affect emotional perception and expression and the more subtle aspects of communication. We also now realise that FTD often progresses much more slowly than older textbooks may suggest, thus having affected family communication and interactions in an insidious way often for years before a diagnosis is clarified. This makes it difficult for family members to distinguish between 'the person they used to know' and 'the person changed by dementia'.

Each marital and family relationship has their own history, and here Gina describes a 'bickering marriage' and says the relationship was 'inequitable'. Family relationships can be complex, and some parents may turn to their children to gain support and understanding of the behaviour of their spouse, the other parent. In this case, Gina was seeking agreement and support from her daughters in the bickering with her husband, which would have been heightened when BvFTD arrived to make him less acquiescent or compromising. The arrival of the dementia can also be seen in the context of the stage of the family's development: in this example, around a time when the daughters left home, became independent and moved away. There may always have been a need for the daughters to distance themselves and leave the parents to get on with their 'bickering', perhaps also re-evaluating which of them was in more need of backing up and supporting in the marital power struggles, leading to the mother feeling hurt, abandoned and grieving the lost closeness and support.

Summary
Considering these dynamics in the context and arrival of a dementia, such underlying issues may become heightened, and the emotional and relational consequences are increased. The long-term consequences can become engrained to a point where families may need additional support in order to overcome these and find a constructive joint approach to living with dementia, or to grieve and heal after the person with dementia has died.

ADMIRAL NURSE ADVICE

Tom Rose, Admiral Nurse Clinical Lead,
St Barnabas Hospice, Lincoln

Carer isolation

Gina describes a very challenging situation when her husband's behaviour started to change. Not only did she have to cope with her own reactions and thoughts about what was happening, but she also had to deal with challenging emotions from her daughters. Gina talks about the previously close relationship she had with her daughters when, it might be imagined, she provided them with emotional support. When the time came for her to need *their* emotional support, Gina found it lacking, leaving her feeling increasingly isolated and estranged from her wider family. Coupled with her daughters' accusations that she wasn't trying hard enough to make their father well, that must have felt very upsetting for Gina. Family carers often expect other people to be supportive of them and to be 'in their corner', yet many family carers (81%) report feeling isolated and alone due to their caring role, and worried about the impact their caring role has on family relationships (Carers UK 2021).

As an Admiral Nurse, it is recognised that Gina needs support in the situation she finds herself in. She needs help to understand the changes she sees in her husband. Providing early support for family carers of a person with dementia can help in avoiding some of the health risks family carers can experience, such as depression. Timely intervention can increase a family carer's resilience for the future by making plans and building stronger support, whether this is in the home or in considering other options, such as respite care. It would also increase the opportunity for Gina to maintain her social connections and engage with her daughters.

Family challenges

Feelings of denial and avoidance, as seen in Gina's daughters, are not uncommon. Family members can feel a sense of loss before the physical death of the person with dementia (see Chapter 7). Gina describes how her daughters found it difficult to accept and adjust to their father's diagnosis, and how they disbelieved what she was telling them. The Admiral Nurse would have been able to help in this situation by exploring each family member's understanding of the changes in the person with dementia and how this was affecting their relationships.

Feeling as though you are standing on ever-shifting ground can add to the perception of a lack of understanding from those around us, and the feelings of uncertainty, anxiety and frustration this generates can be overwhelming. Understanding such changes can help families affected by dementia to maintain relationships. Vital in this is also the need to support Gina's husband in expressing his perspectives about family relationships. How does he perceive his changing role and responsibilities in the family from the past, in the present and in the future?

Changing relationships and roles

Our relationship with others helps to inform our perceptions of situations and the challenges some of these bring. Reinhard has mentioned that when people who are not involved on a very regular basis in the care of a person with dementia and able to see and discuss any changes, this can often cause friction with regular family carers and perspectives may clash. Describing a person with dementia as being 'on their best behaviour' when others visit is not an uncommon observation from the closest carer. This is partly true, in so much that Gina's husband may be trying to maintain the historical format of his relationship with his daughters, where certain boundaries or expected behaviours are maintained. This is in contrast to his relationship with his wife, which, although more volatile, also allows him more freedom for outward expressions of thoughts and feelings.

Relationships change as dementia advances: one person often takes on a greater caring role and so the relationship between the couple, whether spousal or parent/child, has to be 'renegotiated'. How people deal with this change and confront loss can affect the future of a relationship. Family relationships can sometimes become strained and fractured, especially if there is disagreement about the best way forward. There can also be expectations within families about familial duty to care or a feeling of it being a moral failure to ask for external help. As Reinhard has suggested, it sounds as though Gina's daughters were struggling to come to terms with the changes in their father. Whether they were struggling with understanding or accepting the diagnosis is unclear, but a fear of loss can be a powerful driver of feelings and actions. Instead of supporting Gina, her daughters seemed to seek an alternative and less distressing reason for the changes in their father. The effect of this resulted in Gina's perception that her daughters blamed her for something that was not in anyone's control.

Past relationships

Gina tells us of her turbulent relationship with her husband over the years. She speaks of dealing with behaviours that are now deemed excusable because of the diagnosis of dementia, even though this was a continuation of previous issues in their relationship. She asks why she should now accept difficult elements of their relationship simply because of his dementia? Gina is right in that we shouldn't assume that such difficulties are due to a person's dementia. Some difficulties may not be attributable to someone's dementia (known as diagnostic overshadowing). While dementia may be a contributory factor, a person's previous personality, history and relationships are all factors to consider. Historically, Gina and her husband's marital relationship had been at times complicated and fractious, and it is this that is carried through into their relationship now.

It should not be assumed that a person early in the diagnosis of dementia is unable to consider and reflect on their relationships with those around them. It can help to explore with Gina and her husband what their previous relationship had been like, what had been the strengths and what had caused friction. This would allow a discussion about how the presence of dementia may have altered their relationship and pose some questions that would explore and share each of their perceptions. Post-retirement and post-diagnosis, were their values and perceptions fundamentally the same? Did Gina feel that the burden of care was too much to manage in a difficult relationship or did she see this as a way to display affection for her husband? Did her husband see Gina's support as an obligation of the relationship or a situation neither asked for but still found themselves in? What value did her husband place on Gina's support? With the presence of BvFTD, what challenges were there for him in conceptualising and expressing this? These are all questions to be explored in relationship counselling.

Relationship balance

Dementia has altered the balance of the relationship for Gina, her husband and their daughters. It may be that Gina's daughters were not able to recognise the impact that caring was having on their mother and the level of support and care their father needed. This lack of understanding may have been a barrier to a more honest conversation about their mother's needs as a carer and their father's needs arising from his dementia.

It is not uncommon for people with BvFTD to display signs of apathy or unconcern about people and events around them. Coupled with disinhibition in behaviour and language, this could exacerbate the previous relationship difficulties.

Reasoning and judgement may become more difficult as dementia progresses. However, this doesn't mean that family carers should 'soak up' hostility and challenges without the opportunity to express their own views or seek ways to mitigate this. As her husband's dementia progresses and his needs change, it is important to understand what Gina's needs are, her perspectives on her caring role and how she might continue to offer support to her husband. Enabling Gina to explore the historical and current relationship with her husband, including the acceptability of behaviours and how she has dealt with this in the past, will enable her to put into place strategies and to set boundaries in the present.

REFERENCES

Alzheimer's Society (2016) 'Over half of people fear dementia diagnosis, 62 per cent think it means "life is over".' Accessed on 4/7/2022 at www.alzheimers.org.uk/news/2018-05-29/over-half-people-fear-dementia-diagnosis-62-cent-think-it-means-life-over.

Carers UK (2021) '10 facts about loneliness and caring in the UK for Loneliness Awareness Week.' Accessed on 5/5/2022 at www.carersuk.org/news-and-campaigns/news/10-facts-about-loneliness-and-caring-in-the-uk-for-loneliness-awareness-week#_ftnref2.

RESOURCES AND FURTHER READING

Sass, C., Griffiths, A.W., Shoesmith, E., Charura, D. and Nicholson, P. (2021) 'Delivering effective counselling for people with dementia and their families: Opportunities and challenges.' *Counselling and Psychotherapy Research 22*, 1, 175–186. doi:10.1002/capr.12421.

Dementia UK
AFTER A DIAGNOSIS OF DEMENTIA: CHANGING
RELATIONSHIPS AND ROLES

www.dementiauk.org/wp-content/uploads/2020/08/changing-relationships-and-roles.pdf

AFTER A DIAGNOSIS OF DEMENTIA: UNDERSTANDING
AND CHALLENGING STIGMA AND DISCRIMINATION

www.dementiauk.org/wp-content/uploads/2020/08/Understanding-and-challenging-stigma-and-discrimination-1.pdf

Living Together with Dementia
The Tavistock Relationships 'Living Together with Dementia' pro-gramme aims to improve the quality of life and mental health of couples living together with dementia.

https://tavistockrelationships.org/therapeutic-help/living-together-with-dementia

CHAPTER 7

'I feel as though I am going mad'

OVERWHELMING GRIEF

Christine Reddall

My eldest daughter, Anna, was diagnosed with a behavioural variant of frontotemporal dementia aged 37. It took 12 months to correctly diagnose her. She is married with two young sons, but due to her severe behaviour issues, she can no longer live at home. She lived with me and my husband for a while, but her husband felt it would be best if she was placed in a nursing home. I visit her most days, and the pain of watching her deteriorate is unbearable. I feel as though I am encased in a huge black cloud. I expected to feel sad, but the longer the time goes on, the worse I feel. We were told she could live approximately two to five years more with the condition, but the doctors couldn't be more specific. It is now two years since she was diagnosed and the changes in her are massive. The disease seems to be picking away at her brain; more and more of her is disappearing. Just when I think I have seen the worst, another horrid symptom appears.

Most people don't want to see their loved one die, and I hate myself for voicing this, but I wish Anna would die. I feel so guilty that I feel this way, but I am finding it unbearable watching her go through this. I just feel totally overwhelmed and I really don't understand why I am not coping better. I feel so alone, even though I am surrounded by family and friends. I feel lonely inside.

There are so many things that I haven't even told my family about because it's scary and embarrassing. Anna's behaviours are so bizarre that I don't think my friends really believe me when I tell them. I know they struggle to ask me how she is; I can hear it in their voices. Many of my family have stopped visiting Anna as they can't deal with seeing her how she is.

I feel as though I am going mad. My thought processes are all over the place and I am unable to concentrate on anything. I try to read or watch the TV, but I can't follow the plot. I feel on edge all the time as if on constant alert, and I am attached to my mobile phone in case Anna needs me. I panic if it is out of my sight. I am frightened all the time that something might happen and I won't get to her in time. If I go out with friends, I feel unsettled and just want to go home in case the phone rings.

I am not usually an angry person and respect the staff working in care homes as I know their job is not easy. However, I find myself getting so angry at times, especially if the caregivers don't dress Anna nicely, or if they haven't wiped her face after eating.

I am tired, but not just from lack of sleep; it is more like a constant dull feeling. When able to sleep, I now seem to grind my teeth, which is keeping my husband awake as well. I am also suffering from indigestion and I get up most nights to get some medicine. Tears come easily, even over silly little things. I was in a shop the other day, trying to find some pyjamas for Anna. I found a pretty pair, but they didn't have her size on the rail. I asked a shop assistant if they had a bigger size, and when she said no, I burst into tears. I have told the doctor how I am feeling but he just says I am grieving, and it is to be expected.

SPECIALIST COMMENTARY

Dr Kirsten Moore, Senior Research Fellow, National Ageing Research Institute, Victoria, Australia

The unspoken story of grief and loss

Christine's story describes an intense and difficult struggle with grief while caring for her daughter who has dementia. Grief is universal; we will all experience it at some time in our lives, and it is a natural reaction to the death or loss of someone close or important to us. Although we all experience grief, expectations and norms about how we respond and react to grief are shaped by our culture and religion. However, grief is also an individual experience that is as unique as each journey of living with dementia. Grief can be expressed and experienced in many ways and can impact all aspects of our life – emotionally, physically, socially and spiritually. For some, the destruction of our 'assumptive world' – the way we think our world should be – can lead us to question our faith and beliefs. Christine highlights the diversity of these grief reactions including impacts on social relationships, loss of sleep, anger, confusion, loneliness, anxiety, feeling dull and teary. She highlights physical symptoms including digestive problems and teeth grinding.

Changes in the way we think about grief

Previously, theories suggested that grief involved a set of emotions such as sadness, denial and anger that you needed to work through to process grief. However, our thinking has changed, and grief is often now described as an oscillation: alternating between emotions and experiences that may become less intense or less frequent as time passes. Small things, such as that mentioned by Christine, can provide a powerful trigger for intense emotions and can appear to come from nowhere. Most people learn to adapt to losses and manage their grief with support from their family and friends and sometimes other community organisations and religious groups. Some people who are struggling with grief may benefit from professional support and counselling to help them process their thoughts and feelings.

Grief while caring for someone with dementia

Between 47 and 71 per cent of family carers of people with dementia experience grief and around 20 per cent experience significant complicated grief after their relative's death (Chan *et al.* 2013). During the course of dementia, family and friend carers often feel that dementia has substantially altered the person they used to know. Many losses can occur after a diagnosis of dementia. Reduced communication and the person no longer recognising the carer can substantially alter the nature of their relationship. Spouses may feel their future together, such as retirement and travel, has been taken away, and adult children caring for a parent often explain that their roles have reversed and they are now guardians to their parent. People describe not being able to share problems, reminisce or seek advice from the person with dementia. Spouses may feel that transfer to a care home signifies the end of their marriage. Family carers may also experience other personal losses as they give up employment, socialising and interests to support their relative or friend with dementia.

Grief in dementia can be complex due to the nature of dementia, with gradual deterioration over many years. Family carers may feel they have learned to accept one loss when they are faced with something new to adapt to. This can be very taxing on the carer, who may feel there is no respite from needing to adapt to loss. As this grief occurs in the context of demands on the carer's time, they may not feel they have the energy or time to process emotions in the midst of day-to-day pressures.

In our research, we spoke to 150 family carers of people with dementia in England and Wales (Moore *et al.* 2020). We found that those who felt supported by their social network to maintain their health had less intense grief than those who didn't feel supported. We found that women had higher levels of grief than men. Unsurprisingly, those who reported that the closeness of their relationship with the person with dementia had declined since the diagnosis of dementia also showed higher grief levels.

Recognising grief in dementia

One of the challenges of supporting grieving family carers is that their social network may not recognise they are grieving and may not offer the support they would have provided if a death had occurred. Talking about death is a taboo topic, and dementia is also stigmatised; finding a supportive listener can be difficult. Family carers may not feel it is legitimate to grieve someone who is still with them from day to day. Kenneth Doka (1999) called this *disenfranchised* grief as people do not recognise that a loss has occurred. Family carers may no longer want to watch their relative declining and feel that their relative would never have wanted to live with advanced dementia. This can lead to feelings of guilt as it contradicts efforts to cherish and appreciate that their relative is still here with them. It is important that these complex feelings are acknowledged and to know that these emotions are common and reasonable in the context of dementia.

Grief, end-of-life care and death

The losses experienced through the course of dementia mean that family carers are not only anticipating loss but are experiencing loss in the here and now. However, anticipatory grief can occur as the carer may be uncertain about how dementia will progress and how severe it will become. It is likely that educating family carers about the typical progression of dementia and that good-quality care and symptom management can enable a comfortable death may help alleviate their fears and enable them to feel more confident about the future. Informing family carers of the unclear prognosis of dementia can be helpful in enabling them to hold this uncertainty and reduce expectations of knowing when the time will come.

As family carers process grief during the progression of dementia, many expect that death will be a relief. While many family carers do feel relief when their relative dies, they can also experience a fresh new set of loss and emotions. Their importance and role as a carer may have ended, but other aspects of their life may have been put on hold while caring for their relative.

In summary

The experience of grief while caring for someone with dementia can be as intense as grief after death. However, the long duration of dementia and the possible failure to recognise grief by family carers or their support networks can make processing grief and loss more challenging. It is often tied with feelings of guilt by the family carer. Family carers may struggle to find the right support when dealing with loss and concerns about the future. It is important for family carers to acknowledge their feelings of grief and loss, and to be able to find someone who is able to listen to their experiences and provide reassurance and validation of their feelings.

ADMIRAL NURSE ADVICE

Dr Jacqueline Crowther, Helpline Admiral Nurse

Christine appears overwhelmed by many different feelings and emotions. Over time, the Admiral Nurse can facilitate Christine to explore these feelings to help her, arrive at some personal resolution and level of acceptance about what is happening to her daughter due to dementia.

Validating a family carer's emotional response

It is important to acknowledge and validate a family carer's feelings and emotions. The Admiral Nurse would sensitively discuss a family carer's feelings in the context of 'normality'. This will give them the opportunity to think about their feelings, emotions and reaction to the illness, and the things they are finding difficult.

Important in the process of validation is developing a relationship between the Admiral Nurse and the family carer. This will help in identifying those feelings and emotions that are causing the most distress and anxiety and, together, prioritise and address these in order to help them to move forward.

Knowledge and understanding of dementia

A diagnosis of dementia is a life-changing experience for the person themselves and those around them, which has clearly been the case for Christine and her daughter. How the diagnosis of dementia is delivered and what information is shared can affect how and whether people move forward positively with this. It is important to explore a family carer's level of knowledge and understanding about dementia and, in Christine's case, the subtype that Anna has been diagnosed with. Learning more about this, the physiology of the condition and how this is now impacting on Anna's behaviour, might help with Christine's level of understanding, acceptance and planning.

Dementia is recognised as a terminal illness, but many families may not have been made aware of this. Future care planning is recognised as something that can help families living with terminal, life-limiting conditions, including dementia, to think and plan as the disease progresses (see Chapter 5). Engaging in these important conversations and having these and people's wishes documented can make a difference as things change, a person deteriorates and end-of-life approaches, and also help in adjustment and anticipatory grief.

Find your supports

Christine talks of being embarrassed by some of Anna's behaviours and her difficulty in talking to family and friends about this. This is not unusual; family carers can feel uncomfortable sharing feelings and emotions with other family members, usually for fear of worrying or upsetting them. This can lead to people visiting less, which may add to feelings of loneliness and a sense of being overwhelmed by all that is happening. Feeling alone in the situation is difficult; as we see in Christine's case, it is negatively impacting upon her own mental health. It is important to identify any opportunities and people around you who can offer time and space to talk about the feelings and emotions you are experiencing. Peer support is a valuable aspect of dementia care, both for the person with the diagnosis and for family carers. Peer support can help reduce feelings of loneliness, isolation and guilt, and many gain much benefit in connecting with people who are experiencing similar situations.

It is important to understand that feelings such as Christine's are entirely normal in such circumstances. An Admiral Nurse would support you to talk about your sense of grief, specifically anticipatory grief, and the sense of loss often felt when someone close to you is diagnosed with dementia. It is important to monitor your own mental health and, if appropriate, to approach your GP to talk about how you are feeling.

Self-blame

Family carers can often fall into the trap of blaming themselves when things go wrong, or when the care they deliver does not have the outcome they would wish. As we see in Christine's case, she feels anger towards herself when she feels she has not attended to one of Anna's needs as she would have liked. Such feelings of blame are also often felt when a family carer has to relinquish care to formal caregivers. When people with dementia move into a full-time care setting, family carers can often feel frustrated and angry when the person with dementia is not cared for as they would like or as they would do themselves, if able (also see Chapter 15). Family carers do not stop caring when people with dementia move into full-time care; it is more that the role changes. This transition can be very difficult for some and often complicate any feelings of grief. Again, an Admiral Nurse would offer the opportunity to discuss the feelings of anger, normalise them and help family carers to develop strategies to manage or avoid the negative feelings and the impact these have.

Powerlessness

Feelings of powerlessness might be something else that can contribute to feelings of anger and frustration. It is important to enable family carers to talk about their changing situation and feelings as they arise. Family carers find it helpful if they can negotiate becoming a care partner in some way with the formal caregivers within the care facility, thus enabling a continued sense of involvement and influence over care. In Christine's case, this could include her contribution to the development of a care plan for Anna's care. Activities to enable Christine to maintain contact with Anna's care could include things such as the Namaste model of care (Simard 2007) to enable Christine to still feel connected to Anna (see Chapter 16). Developed as a way of supporting and communicating with people with more advanced dementia, Namaste employs activities in communication that use all the senses and enables good quality of life and positive connections when communication is more challenged. Exploring with Christine how she can continue to connect with Anna may help her accept some of the changes she is observing in Anna, combat Christine's sense of powerlessness and have a positive impact on her own mental health.

Self-care

Family carers need time for themselves. To take care of and be kind and compassionate to oneself at such difficult and demanding times is essential for any family carer's wellbeing. Together, the Admiral Nurse and family carer can identify ways to do this, including focusing on all the things they can still do with the person with dementia and reminding themselves of all the things they still do and do well.

In summary, the Admiral Nurse would support Christine using a person-centred, sensitive, supportive and validating approach. It is important to normalise a family carer's feelings and give permission to experience and feel these, even the negative ones. It is important that family carers know that what they are feeling is normal and a common reaction, and, as in Christine's case with Anna, that there will be good days and bad days. The Admiral Nurse will encourage and support Christine to find an outlet for her feelings and emotions. Identifying positive opportunities going forward will enable family carers to continue to see the joy and love in her relationship with the person with dementia, even though this is very different from what either had planned.

REFERENCES

Chan, D., Livingston, G., Jones, L. and Sampson, E.L. (2013) 'Grief reactions in dementia carers: A systematic review.' *International Journal of Geriatric Psychiatry 28*, 1, 1–17. doi:10.1002/gps.3795.

Doka, K.J. (1999) 'Disenfranchised grief.' *Bereavement Care 18*, 3, 37–39. doi:10.1080/02682629908657467.

Moore, K.J., Crawley, S., Vickerstaff, V., Cooper, C., King, M. and Sampson, E.L. (2020) 'Is preparation for end of life associated with pre-death grief in caregivers of people with dementia?' *International Psychogeriatrics 32*, 6, 753–763. doi:10.1017/S1041610220000289.

Simard. J. (2007) *The End-of-Life Namaste Care Program for People with Dementia*. Towson, MD: Health Professions Press.

RESOURCES AND FURTHER READING

James, O. (2008) *Contented Dementia: 24-Hour Wraparound Care for Lifelong Well-Being*. London: Vermilion.

McCurry, S.M. (2006) *When a Family Member Has Dementia: Steps to Becoming a Resilient Caregiver*. Westport, CT: Greenwood World Publishing.

Caring for family or friends with dementia: could these feelings be grief?

This animation has been developed to raise awareness of the grief family and friends may experience while caring for someone with dementia. It has been developed for a wide audience including family and friend carers, along with their friends, family and social network, as well as healthcare professionals and those working with family and friend carers.

www.ucl.ac.uk/psychiatry/research/marie-curie-palliative-care-research-department/research/centre-dementia-palliative-care-23

Dementia UK
GRIEF (INCLUDING ANTICIPATORY GRIEF),
BEREAVEMENT AND LOSS

> www.dementiauk.org/get-support/family-and-carer-support/
> bereavement

Rare Dementia Support
Rare Dementia Support is for everyone affected by or at risk of a rare dementia, to have access to information, tailored support and contact with others affected by similar conditions in a space of mutual respect and understanding.

> www.raredementiasupport.org

together in dementia everyday (tide)
tide is an organisation that gives you the opportunity to meet other carers, to hear and share stories with other carers, to help with the isolation and loneliness many feel.

> www.tide.uk.net

CHAPTER 8

'How does physical ill-health affect people with dementia?'

UNDERSTANDING DELIRIUM

Alfie Jones (pseudonym)

For the past two years, I have suspected that Dad has the early stages of dementia: he is forgetful, repeats things, and gets very muddled with things like the TV remote, his new phone and anything that seems to fall out of his usual routine. He lives alone but copes quite well on the whole. Because he manages fairly well, I only need to call in twice a week to make sure he has food in the house and that he is safe and happy.

I went on holiday for a couple of weeks, so hadn't visited Dad as I would have done, but he said he didn't need any help while I was away. When I got back, I visited him and he was very confused and agitated, and his sitting room and kitchen were in a real mess. When I asked him what had happened, he was upset and said he could see insects everywhere and the place was a mess as he was trying to get rid of them. I looked around the house and could see no evidence of insects, but he kept saying, 'Look, they are everywhere; you must have something wrong with your eyes!'

I managed to calm Dad down and I gave him a cup of tea and a sandwich while I tidied up. However, when I made his sandwich, I noticed that he hadn't touched the food I bought him before I went on holiday, and much of it was now out of date. I also noticed that there was urine on the hall floor near to the toilet door.

Dad didn't look well. He was sweaty and looked frightened, and his memory problems were much worse, and I felt so guilty that I had left him to fend for himself for so long. I was really worried about Dad and didn't know what to do. I wondered whether this was due to a possible worsening of the dementia. I felt guilty I hadn't taken Dad for an assessment sooner, when I first had an inkling that something was wrong – this on top of feeling guilty because I had left him to cope on his own for so long.

On a friend's advice, I called the Admiral Nurse Dementia Helpline, and the nurse advised me to contact the GP as they said Dad may have a physical health problem causing his sudden change in behaviour.

SPECIALIST COMMENTARY

Professor Rowan H. Harwood, Consultant Geriatrician, University of Nottingham/ Nottingham University Hospitals NHS Trust

Unexpected things happening, things going wrong, crises and emergencies are unfortunately common for people with dementia. They are vulnerable to physical illness, falls and loss of usual abilities, side effects of prescription drugs, mental distress, changes in usual family or social support, or in the physical environment or location. When a crisis occurs, families, social care and healthcare professional staff have to work out what is the cause, and what can be done, and often there are several things at once. This will usually require additional support from families or professional health and social care, diagnosis and treatment by a GP, or admission to hospital.

Delirium

Delirium is a sudden onset or worsening of confusion due to a physical illness, injury, operation, drug or drug withdrawal. 'Sudden' means coming on over hours or days. 'Confusion' means that memory, flow of thinking and speech are worse than usual. The person may ramble or flit from topic to topic. A key element is inattentiveness – this means anything from drowsiness or sleeping to inability to focus and distractibility. Delirium fluctuates; it varies from one minute or hour to the next. It is often worse at night.

There may also be delusions or hallucinations. A delusion is a false belief, which is firmly held and cannot be corrected by explanation or reasoning (see also Chapter 10). Delusions in delirium are often paranoid or persecutory, such as a belief that the person is in danger or going to be harmed. The belief is very real to the person who holds it, often intense and frightening. Delusions will often be the cause of agitation, resistance or aggression, which can be seen as a form of self-defence. Hallucinations are usually visions, usually formed, and they include moving animals or people, but may also be bizarre or distorted. Occasionally, hallucinations may be unpleasant feelings on the skin or voices providing a commentary or instructions. Extreme emotions can be felt, such as anxiety, depression, terror or anger. The person may be passive and withdrawn or restless and agitated, or vary between the two. They may become unsteady on their feet or incontinent of urine. Delirium is very variable and changes, so there may be good and worse times. The physical consequences of any underlying illness may also complicate the picture.

What causes delirium?

The cause can be virtually any illness imaginable. Infections are commonest, from a cold or chest infection through to meningitis or other serious internal infections. Worsening of confusion is often attributed to a urinary infection or 'UTI'; although this is possible, urinary infections are over-diagnosed, and in doing so we risk both missing the real cause and misusing antibiotics. The second commonest cause is prescription (or occasionally recreational) drugs: especially morphine-like (opioid) drugs, Parkinson's drugs or other drugs affecting the nervous system. Drug withdrawal can cause delirium, including alcohol, opioids and benzodiazepines. All drugs have minor side effects, which can add up, and simply being on many drugs at once can cause cumulative problems, without us being able to pin it down to a single culprit. Strokes, heart attacks and heart failure, fractures and lung disease can be added to the long list of possible causes. Even conditions such as constipation, pain and lack of sleep are associated with delirium, and may or may not be direct causes in themselves.

Diagnosing delirium

There are two parts to diagnosis: identifying that delirium is present or possible; then finding the cause. Identifying delirium reliably can be hard, even for experienced doctors and nurses, because it is so variable. Many doctors and nurses lack expertise in delirium, so it sometimes gets ignored or misinterpreted. Identifying the cause can be equally difficult – in over half of cases there are multiple possible causes, and in up to a quarter of cases no convincing illness can be found despite a thorough search. This can lead to frustration all round.

Diagnosis depends on a good account of what has happened and what has changed, which often relies on a family member or professional carer. Recently started or stopped drugs are identified as part of the assessment process. The doctor or nurse will examine for attention, sometimes using a test such as reciting days of the week backwards. They may perform a memory test and will ask about delusions and hallucinations, but this is skillful and has to be subtle, as people who are fearful for their safety may not readily reveal what they are thinking. The doctor or nurse will then set about trying to find the cause or causes, using symptoms, examination and blood, urine, X-rays or other tests, as required. This may need hospital admission, which itself is often disruptive and can be distressing. Often, it is practical problems with risky or uncooperative behaviours, or deteriorating physical abilities such as walking, falling or continence that make staying at home impossible.

Treating delirium

Treatment comprises finding and treating the underlying cause. Delirium is sometimes brief and resolves quickly. Unfortunately, it can also be slow and may take several months to get better. So it is also important to give recovery long enough, and try to avoid making big decisions, such as moving to a care home, too soon. We must also try to protect the person from complications, such as injuries from falls, malnutrition, pressures sores, weakness and loss of abilities caused by inactivity. We may use antipsychotic drugs to control delusions and hallucinations, but they are not always effective. Sometimes (such as in alcohol withdrawal, or delirium complicating Parkinson's disease or dementia with Lewy bodies) benzodiazepines, such as lorazepam, can be used with some effect.

In about a fifth of cases, delirium does not resolve despite treatment. Some research indicates that episodes of delirium could be a mechanism through which dementia gets worse (Pereira *et al.* 2021).

Delirium indicates serious ill-health. The biggest risk factors are age, prior dementia, severe illness and injures (such as hip fracture). Up to half of people who have delirium will not survive the next six months, and delirium is very common in people who are dying. However, many people do recover, either to full mental health or to the level of confusion seen before the episode. Delusions, hallucinations and fragile emotions usually settle or pass.

Nowadays, we put a lot of emphasis on preventing delirium. This includes anything to promote general physical health, including vaccination, preventative medication for the heart or bones and falls prevention. We must be very careful in prescribing, trying to avoid a list of high-risk drugs and to minimise the overall number of tablets taken. It is also important to observe for problems when medication is started or stopped. Delirium can be prevented by ensuring that an older person drinks and eats enough, glasses and hearing aids are worn and maintained, they keep mobile, sleep well (without sleeping tablets) and keep mentally stimulated.

Mr Jones and delirium

Did Mr Jones Senior have delirium? There was a change. Alfie had correctly identified that his father probably had dementia: he was forgetful and struggling with complex activities, and it was causing problems in daily life. He was more confused and agitated, and was hallucinating insects. He didn't look well and he was sweaty, which might indicate an infection or other physical illness. Alternatively, pallor and sweating could reflect anxiety (at the insect infestation) and anger (at his son for denying what was obvious to him). At first sight, there was no obvious physical illness, but older people do not always show classical signs of illness, and it is impossible to say that there was none without further assessment and investigation.

The fact that food left by Alfie for his father had been untouched makes me wonder whether Mr Jones's dementia was more severe than had been appreciated. People with dementia rely on familiarity and routine. Attentive, diligent and discreet care from his son will have provided compensation for mental limitations and inabilities. When that help was suddenly no longer available – and everyone needs a break or a holiday sometime – the extent of Mr Jones's limitations could have been laid bare.

That would not have explained the new hallucinations, however. There are two main explanations for hallucinations in this situation. Hallucinations caused by the dementia itself, or delirium. One particular type of dementia, dementia with Lewy bodies (or the related condition, Parkinson's disease dementia), typically has visual hallucinations. They can also sometimes occur in people with Alzheimer's disease or people with poor vision. The sudden onset and severity make delirium the more likely explanation, but this is not definite. Vascular dementia gets worse in 'steps', and the sudden decline can look like delirium. Visual hallucinations are relatively uncommon in vascular dementia, but you learn 'never to say never' in medicine. We might presume that Mr Jones had not been drinking alcohol heavily and suddenly had his supply cut off, but it would be good to ask, discreetly. We should also ask if any other drugs had been stopped or started.

Mr Jones needs a proper and thorough medical and mental state assessment to properly work out what is going on, so that treatable conditions, such as infections, could be treated, and a plan drawn up for how to weather the crisis. His son should be reassured that these things happen; he had provided sterling service over a prolonged time to enable his father to thrive at home and was in no way responsible for the deterioration.

ADMIRAL NURSE ADVICE

Kerry Lyons, Consultant Admiral Nurse – Acute Services, Dementia UK

It is important as a carer not to feel guilty when a sudden change occurs. Living independently with 'usual routines' can be an extremely important aspect to living as well as possible with dementia.

When sudden changes occur, it is important to seek a medical opinion to exclude delirium in the first instance. After the delirium has been treated and resolved then it would be pertinent to raise the concerns with his GP about Mr Jones Senior's problems with his memory that span a longer period. This may result in a referral to a memory assessment service.

Delirium is a treatable condition that often co-exists with dementia. At times, it can be difficult to identify and distinguish between dementia and delirium. This is often due to their symptoms being very similar, and it therefore may not always be picked up immediately or until there has been a significant change in a person's perception of reality and/or a significant change in behaviour.

Delirium can be extremely distressing for both the person with dementia and their carer. Symptoms can often develop slowly or there may be a sudden change in the person's behaviour. Delirium can last days or even months, and when it occurs alongside dementia it can often take the person longer to recover.

Managing the symptoms

As in Mr Jones's case, visual hallucinations are a common symptom, which can be very distressing for both the person with dementia and their carer. The hallucinations lead to an altered sense of reality (see Chapter 9), increasing the person's confusion and often escalating their distress. When a person experiences hallucinations, the main aim would be to support them to feel safe, reduce their distress and try to orientate them to the present. This could be done by listening to the person and validating their feelings of distress. Ask the person what the matter is and/or try to find the sources of their distress. Reassurance of safety should be offered – you may want to try sitting close and holding the person's hand to offer familiarity and comfort. Giving time and explanation using short and simple sentences with a low and non-threatening tone can help the person feel they are listened to and supported. Try to avoid disagreeing with the person; if necessary, use distraction techniques – for example, offer a drink or a snack, engage them in an activity they enjoy – to divert them from any hallucinations or delusional thought process (see Chapter 10).

Sometimes the delirium may be caused or exacerbated by pain, so make sure that the person is not in any physical pain. Start by asking them directly if they are in pain; however, sometimes they may not be able to voice this, so you may need to observe for behaviours that indicate the presence of pain, such as holding or rubbing the painful part of the body (see Chapter 16). Ensure medication is taken as prescribed, and that pain experienced is appropriately managed – seek help if in doubt.

Ensure that their usual communication aids are used and that any glasses or hearing devices are clean and in working order. Orientate the person to the time, date and their space (use photos and familiar objects to anchor the person to their usual reality). Assist the person to 'way-find' – for example, route to the toilet, bathroom or bedroom; this might involve directional signs or labelling each of the doors. Keep the environment as familiar, calm and settled as possible; low noise and ambient lighting may help to alleviate a person's distress.

Offer diet and fluids to maintain their nutrition and hydration, and remember to be flexible. For example, if the person does not want to drink, you could offer 'wet' foods such as yoghurts and soups to increase their fluid intake.

Aiding recovery

Re-establishing the person's routine as they recover from the underlying condition that brought about the delirium is important. Offer them familiar anchors to re-engage with their usual activities, ideally including things that the person enjoys. Reintroduce activities gradually as the person's health allows, such as going for a walk or visiting liked and familiar places. In addition, you could try to ensure a good wake–sleep pattern, reducing the risk of end-of-the-day confusion (known as sundowning – see Chapter 13) by:

- limiting daytime naps

- reducing caffeine and alcohol consumption

- setting the scene for night by closing curtains

- introducing bedtime routines to mark the transition of day to night.

Try to look around the person's environment with 'fresh eyes'. Look for objects that may be misinterpreted and create additional distress.

This may include shiny or reflective floors which the person may misinterpret as a pool of water or an unsafe surface to walk on. A dressing gown hanging on a door may be misinterpreted as another person, and a reflection of themselves in a mirror may be mistaken for an intruder.

Mr Jones Senior

Sometimes poor dietary or fluid intake may cause or exacerbate delirium, so it is important to monitor what the person eats and drinks over time. In the case of Mr Jones Senior, it would appear that he was not eating the food his son left when he went on holiday.

Alfie noticed that there was urine on the hall floor when he visited his father, and this may have been an indication that he could not find the toilet or couldn't make it in time, or it could be evidence of incontinence, possibly due to an infection. Constipation and urinary infections can be a cause or consequence of delirium; in either case, this will need to be prevented or treated.

Alfie felt guilty that he hadn't sought help for his father earlier and hadn't realised that his father's needs had increased until he went on holiday and found his father had not coped without his care and support. As Admiral Nurses, we often come across these feelings of guilt and worry that the family member is not doing enough to support the person with dementia. It is important not to be too hard on yourself as a carer and to remember that you are doing the best that you can do. It is important to recognise when you need additional help to prevent distress or a crisis. Family carers also need to seek early support, advice and guidance when facing some of the changes that can be experienced when someone close has dementia. This is often a new experience for all parties, so it is not surprising specialist dementia advice and support is needed. Listen to yourself as a carer and remember that you know the person best of all and will intuitively know what helps to make them feel safe, so trust in your instincts.

REFERENCE

Pereira, J.V.B., Aung Thein, M.Z., Nitchingham, A. and Caplan, G.A. (2021) 'Delirium in older adults is associated with development of new dementia: A systematic review and meta-analysis.' *International Journal of Geriatric Psychiatry 36*, 7, 993–1003. doi:10.1002/gps.5508.

RESOURCES AND FURTHER READING
Royal College of Psychiatrists: Delirium

Information for anyone who has experienced delirium, knows someone with delirium or is looking after people with delirium.

www.rcpsych.ac.uk/mental-health/problems-disorders/delirium

Dementia UK
UNDERSTANDING CHANGES IN DEMENTIA:
DELIRIUM (SUDDEN CONFUSION)

www.dementiauk.org/get-support/understanding-changes-in-dementia/delirium

CHAPTER 9

'I thought dementia was just about memory loss'

HALLUCINATIONS

JACK AND CAROLINE WORTH (PSEUDONYMS)

Jack

I first noticed the problem while driving. It was for a flash of a second, as if a cloud had surrounded my brain and made it difficult for me to figure out the lane markings on the road. The lines seem to merge together, and I wasn't sure which lane I ought to be in. I could see the lorries clearly, but were they close behind or far away? I panicked and left the motorway as quickly as I could, though fortunately I got home safely. I put this down to being tired from driving a long distance that day, but the panic left me with a dreadful feeling in my stomach. The problems then slowly began to get worse.

I then found myself tripping up at home. Sometimes there was a step...but sometimes there wasn't; I could never be sure. It was as if my brain was being tricked. Being a retired electrical engineer, fiddling with circuit boards was my favourite pastime. I could spend hours connecting and reconnecting them for my various projects. However, it became harder to do this and took me forever to fathom the circuits, so that I eventually had to give up.

It was my wife, Caroline, who noticed that I was walking differently. She said I always seemed in a hurry and felt that was the reason I might be falling sometimes. I couldn't explain to her that I couldn't stop myself from walking like this, even if I wanted to. She insisted that

I see the doctor, who examined me and said he thought I had signs of Parkinson's, but he couldn't be sure so he referred me to a neurologist. This is when things seemed to get serious. The neurologist made me walk, turn, do some exercises, and sent me for a special scan and made me do lots of tests on counting, drawing, remembering things, repeating words, reading, writing. His tests seemed endless, but he was very thorough, which was sort of reassuring in a way. Drawing was now particularly difficult for me, which surprised Caroline as only a few years ago I had drawn the plans for our house renovations. Now I couldn't even manage a simple line drawing for the neurologist. The doctor said he suspected I could have a type of dementia, which really shocked us. We always thought people with dementia forget things, and my memory wasn't too bad at this point. He made me an appointment for a brain scan. We went back for the results of the scan where I was told I had a type of dementia called dementia with Lewy bodies.

That was two years ago now, and things are very different... I'll let Caroline tell how she sees things from her perspective.

Caroline

Today is a good day, but not all days are as good as this. Since we came to know Jack's problems were down to this dementia with Lewy bodies, life has been a roller coaster. It has been difficult for both of us really. I have found it particularly hard to adjust to the way Jack can change from day to day, or even from morning to the evening on the same day. We had friends come over yesterday, and Jack was amazing. He knew their names and chatted away over some old, shared memories, and we were all pleased. But that evening, after they had gone, it was a different story. Jack seemed so confused. In fact, he couldn't recognise where he was in our house, and it was so scary to watch him look around in a panicked way as if he didn't know where he was. These periods of confusion are happening more often, and it fills me with dread to think, 'What if he doesn't recognise me one day?' It is difficult to go anywhere or plan anything as I cannot predict how Jack is going to react to things. It is as if he is a different person from one day to another. I am slowly learning to cope with this, but I feel I cannot leave him alone at home even now. What if he gets into one of his confused states and comes to harm?

Jack also started seeing 'visions' in our back garden a few months back. Initially, I thought he had mistaken some of the bushes in the garden, thinking perhaps, at first glance, they were people. But then one day he pointed at the floor in the lounge and said he could see small dwarves. He would try to shout at them and chase them away, getting himself wound up. I tried to pass it off and make him realise these are not real, but then he only got angry with me and accused me of trying to make him look 'stupid'. The doctor says these visions are also part of his condition, but sometimes he gets so stressed that these people are trying to take over our house that no amount of explanation or reassurance seems to calm him down.

SPECIALIST COMMENTARY

Dr Malarvizhi Babu Sandilyan, Consultant in Old Age Psychiatry, and Professor Tom Dening, Professor of Dementia Research

Dementia with Lewy bodies (DLB) is the second most common cause of dementia in older people (Walker *et al.* 2015). Like other types of dementia, it is a progressive brain disorder causing cognitive decline enough to cause a significant interference in complex activities of daily living. The characteristic features of DLB are said to be cognitive fluctuations (what Caroline describes as Jack's level of confusion being different from day to day), visual hallucinations and Parkinsonism (symptoms similar to those seen in Parkinson's disease, such as tremors, bradykinesia (generally slow movements), rigidity, shuffling gait, etc.).

Cognitive problems

People with DLB present with distinctive neurocognitive and behavioural features compared with those affected with other types of dementia, and they also show similar symptoms to those seen in Parkinson's disease. DLB affects general cognitive functions such as memory, language and planning. However, compared with Alzheimer's disease, someone with DLB has more difficulty with visuospatial abilities – that is, a person's ability to recognise where they are in relation to the environment around them. These visuospatial difficulties can lead to symptoms such as missing the chair when sitting down, tripping on stairs/carpets or misjudging distances while driving.

Here, Jack describes his developing problems that led to a diagnosis of dementia – in his case, dementia with Lewy bodies. Note that some of his early symptoms were not related to typical memory loss (as characteristically seen in Alzheimer's disease); instead, he was having problems with judging space and distance. Jack also finds it difficult with his hobby working on circuit boards, something that requires attention, visual perceptual skills and planning. Problems in areas such as spatial awareness, depth/distance perception, object relationships in space and the person are collectively termed as visuoperceptual difficulties and they are a prominent and early feature in DLB (McKeith *et al.* 2020).

Fluctuations

What Caroline reports as Jack's changing level of confusion is termed 'cognitive fluctuation', which is a commonly recognised feature of DLB. In fact, it is one of the core diagnostic features in the diagnosis of DLB (McKeith *et al.* 2017). It refers to a person's change in alertness, attention and cognition, and can include periods of reduced attention, staring spells and confusion, which last from seconds to hours. Changes in cognitive function are also common and can alternate from being very significant to near normal functioning. Family carers may also report that the person is 'inattentive' or 'vacant' for times lasting from a few seconds to minutes. This can be challenging for family carers as the person may appear unpredictable and changeable. Although minor day-to-day variations in a person's confusion can occur in all types of dementia, the severity and variation between the best and worst times are most marked in DLB. Sometimes, the fluctuations are so dramatic that it appears that the person has delirium due to a physical illness.

Visual hallucinations

Jack reports seeing people who are not actually there, a symptom called an hallucination (a perception without a stimulus) and as he sees (as opposed to hearing, smelling or feeling) them, so they are called visual hallucinations. Though common in some other psychiatric and neurological conditions, visual hallucinations are one of the core features of DLB and can cause high levels of both carer stress and distress for the person with DLB. They can vary from simple hallucinations, such as seeing a flash or geometric shape, to well-formed ones that represent people or animals, as in Jack's case. It may be that hallucinations result from altered function of the chemical transmitter acetylcholine in the brain. Sometimes rivastigmine, which is a drug often used in Alzheimer's disease, may help as a treatment. Antipsychotic drugs can also be used to treat hallucinations, but people with DLB are very susceptible to their side effects, so they are generally best avoided or, if necessary, only prescribed by a specialist.

Other symptoms

DLB may cause movement symptoms similar to those in Parkinson's disease, such as shuffling, a short-stepped gait, reduced arm swing while walking, reduced facial expressions, rigidity, tremors and slowness in movements (bradykinesia). These can cause problems with walking, turning, getting up from a low chair or out of bed, and may even lead to frequent falls.

Another characteristic symptom of DLB is known as REM (rapid eye movement) sleep behaviour disorder. REM sleep is a phase of sleeping in which dreams often occur, and the person's eyes move around rapidly behind their closed eyelids (Chan *et al.* 2018). Normally, during REM sleep, the person's limbs do not move as their muscle tone is absent, but in DLB this arrangement becomes disturbed. As a result, the person may appear to be enacting their dreams and moving around vigorously in their sleep. This can be to the extent where they injure themselves or their bed partner, and they also may appear very distressed.

There are a lot of other symptoms that may occur in DLB. These include mood changes, such as depression and anxiety, delusions, apathy and autonomic dysfunction – that is, problems with automatic bodily functions, which can include constipation, incontinence of urine, feeling dizzy on standing up (postural hypotension) and day-time sleepiness.

Brain changes

DLB is characterised by presence of 'Lewy bodies' (named after Friedrich Lewy who first described them in 1912). Lewy bodies are also typical of Parkinson's disease, and the two diseases do share many similarities. People with Parkinson's disease often develop dementia eventually, too. Lewy bodies are microscopic deposits in the brain, formed mainly of a protein called alpha-synuclein. It is not clear whether Lewy bodies cause damage to the brain or whether they are simply markers of damage or even part of the brain's response to heal itself. However, where they are distributed in the brain affects the symptoms that occur. For example, if the Lewy bodies are found mainly in the cerebral cortex (the thin layer covering the outer surface of the brain), then dementia is more likely, but if the Lewy bodies are mainly in the base of the brain, this tends to produce Parkinson's disease.

Treatment

Cholinesterase inhibitors, commonly known as anti-dementia drugs (donepezil, rivastigmine and galantamine), which are largely used in Alzheimer's disease, appear to be effective in DLB, too. They can not only improve a person's cognitive performance but also may be effective in treating delusions and hallucinations. Medical treatment of neuropsychiatric features such as depression, anxiety and psychosis involve antidepressants and antipsychotics, although (as mentioned above) the latter are associated with serious side effects and are best avoided if possible. Treating DLB often works well if there is close liaison with a Parkinson's specialist. This can often help with the management of any medications for the symptoms of Parkinsonism.

As with other forms of dementia, psychological and social support to the person with the diagnosis and to their families is crucially important. This includes providing sufficient information about the symptoms and problems associated with DLB.

Summary

Dementia with Lewy bodies is a common type of dementia and can present with a wide range of symptoms, some of which overlap with those of Parkinson's disease. It is caused by excessive deposits of abnormal proteins in areas of the brain, which can precede the actual clinical symptoms by several years. Treatment is multifaceted in this complex condition but includes psychosocial support as well as medical treatment aimed at improving cognitive performance and reducing the burden of motor symptoms and any associated psychiatric symptoms.

ADMIRAL NURSE ADVICE

Rachel Thompson, Consultant Admiral Nurse

Dementia with Lewy bodies can be particularly challenging for both the person with the diagnosis and family carers due to the complexity and unpredictability of symptoms. Both Jack and Caroline highlight some of the frequent distress experienced as a result of visual hallucinations, changes in visual perception, Parkinson's symptoms and fluctuations in cognition. Adjusting to a diagnosis of any long-term condition can be challenging, but the experience of those with DLB has been shown to be particularly difficult and can sometimes lead to a lower quality of life than in other types of dementia. It is therefore essential that families are supported in understanding the condition, managing symptoms, adjusting to change and accessing practical support and treatment.

Education and skills training

It is recommended that people with dementia and their families are offered psychoeducation and skills training, including information about the type of dementia that has been diagnosed. There is often support available from local services and/or voluntary sector organisations that is either delivered in a group setting or individualised. However, such support is often focused on the most common symptoms of dementia, such as memory loss, disorientation in time and changes in a person's ability to function, as opposed to the characteristic symptoms faced by people with DLB.

Tailored approach

In order to meet the different needs of a family affected by dementia, an approach that is tailored to that situation may often be required.

This can involve a range of interventions and activities which may be provided individually, as a couple (where the person with dementia is able to contribute) or with a wider family group. Providing an opportunity for both the person with dementia and the family carer to have separate time to share concerns, as well as explore solutions together, may be particularly helpful. In DLB, this is particularly relevant as people with a diagnosis of this type of dementia often retain insight (awareness) into their condition, particularly in the earlier stages.

Assessment

An assessment includes exploring the mental and physical health needs of both the person and their family caregiver, including any other illnesses in addition to the dementia and their treatments. The Admiral Nurse will assess the needs of both the person with dementia and their family caregiver; this will help to ascertain their different perspectives about the condition and its impact on them as individuals as well as on their relationship. This will include exploring each person's understanding of the different symptoms and knowledge about disease progression. Symptoms can be complex and numerous, so it is useful to find out which are most troublesome, noting this may differ for the person with dementia and their caregiver. As we see in this case, Jack's main concerns appear to be his loss of function and loss of independence, whereas Caroline is concerned about the cognitive fluctuations, distressing hallucinations and uncertainty about the future.

A comprehensive assessment often elicits further issues that families may be less aware of. People with DLB can experience high levels of apathy, anxiety and depression, as well as hallucinations, delusions, sleep disturbance and Parkinsonism. These can have a negative impact on family carers who may have an increased risk of anxiety and depression as a result. It is important that any symptoms of anxiety and depression are assessed so that appropriate psychological and/or pharmacological treatments can be accessed.

As mentioned earlier, people with DLB often retain insight into their condition in the earlier stages. As we see in Jack's case, change in memory was not his main symptom. Jack's decreased functional abilities, such as increased falls, difficulty with drawing and engaging in his previous pastime of 'fiddling with circuit boards', were his main areas of concern and frustration. Loss of previous skills or abilities can lead to a lowering of confidence and sense of purpose, leaving people with dementia feeling they are no longer able to contribute in a meaningful way.

Peer support

Jack could be offered the opportunity to air his feelings about these changes, help to think about his personal strengths and then explore activities that could enable him to maintain a sense of purpose and fulfilment. Similarly, sharing experiences with his peers could be particularly helpful to Jack, so encouragement to engage with local face-to-face or online groups for people with a diagnosis of dementia could be considered. Peer support groups may be available through his local services, cognitive stimulation groups, day centres, dementia cafés or DEEP groups (Dementia Engagement and Empowerment Project).

Hallucinations and fluctuating symptoms

The changes or fluctuations in symptoms and abilities from day to day, or even within the same day, can be difficult to manage. Such fluctuations are frequently cited as a source of stress for family carers and can have a major impact on their wellbeing and ability to continue in their caring role. Caroline describes the distress caused by Jack's 'visions'. What Caroline describes as visions are hallucinations and changes in Jack's visual perception, and these can be very stressful for family carers of people with DLB.

Psychoeducational support is a structured approach to provide knowledge about various aspects of an illness and its treatment, through emotional and motivational aspects to enable people and their families to better understand, cope with and manage the illness. Such an approach would help increase Caroline's understanding of the hallucinations and support her to develop responses that may help reduce associated distress – for example, encouraging Caroline not to question or challenge the hallucinations but instead offer Jack reassurance and encourage distraction if possible. People with DLB dementia can be supported to challenge their own hallucinations if enough insight is retained.

Managing risk

Part of the assessment would also consider any possible risks for both the person with dementia and the family caregiver, to address any immediate or longer-term concerns. For example, Caroline expresses concern about Jack's risk of falling and injury if she ever has to leave him at home alone. There may be strategies that would take a more positive risk-taking approach, which can support the person with dementia to be as independent as possible while minimising any unnecessary risk. This may involve the use of assistive technology to monitor Jack's activity and reduce anxiety for Caroline. Alternatively, Caroline could seek support from friends and family or home respite or befriending services. Other areas of assessment may include financial and legal issues such as benefits, Lasting Power of Attorney, advance care planning and accessing practical and informal support, such as discussions about planning for the future while Jack is still able. Much of this is covered in other sections of this book.

Due to increased physical needs along with unpredictable and distressing symptoms in DLB, people may withdraw from social networks and become increasingly isolated. Jack and Caroline may benefit from psychosocial support (the support given to help meet the mental, emotional, social and spiritual needs of people with dementia and their families) in maintaining health and wellbeing, such as taking part in physical activities and social engagement, as well as developing positive strategies to manage stress, anxiety and low mood.

Medication management is also particularly important in DLB as some pharmacological treatments, such as Parkinson's medication, can lead to worsening of other symptoms, such as hallucinations. Other medications should also be used with caution, including antipsychotic and anticholinergic medications which may be used to treat other symptoms or conditions. It is important to seek advice and support regarding some medications, and the Admiral Nurse could support this by liaising with the doctor who prescribes Jack's medicines for his DLB.

In summary

People diagnosed with DLB, as with other types of dementia, live within relational context with other family members, friends and communities, so a relationship- and/or family-centred approach to care and support is essential. Families affected by DLB are faced with particularly difficult challenges due to the condition's complex physical, cognitive and psychosocial needs, and as such may require tailored support in managing and addressing these specific needs. Admiral Nurses, with a specialist knowledge of dementia, can support families in understanding and managing the particularly challenging symptoms of DLB, which may help reduce feelings of frustration and isolation and support families in feeling better prepared.

REFERENCES

Chan, P.C., Lee, H.H., Hong, C.T., Hu, C.J. and Wu, D. (2018) 'REM sleep behavior disorder (RBD) in dementia with Lewy bodies (DLB).' *Behavioural Neurology 2018*, 9421098. doi:10.1155/2018/9421098.

McKeith, I.G., Boeve, B.F., Dickson, D.W., Halliday, G. *et al.* (2017) 'Diagnosis and management of dementia with Lewy bodies: Fourth consensus report of the DLB Consortium.' *Neurology* 89, 1, 88–100. doi:10.1212/WNL.0000000000004058.

McKeith, I.G., Ferman, T.J., Thomas, A.J., Blanc, F. *et al.* (2020) 'Research criteria for the diagnosis of prodromal dementia with Lewy bodies.' *Neurology 94*, 17, 743–755. doi:10.1212/WNL.0000000000009323.

Walker, Z., Possin, K.L., Boeve, B.F. and Aarsland, D. (2015) 'Lewy body dementias.' *Lancet 386*, 10004, 1683–1697. doi:10.1016/S0140-6736(15)00462-6.

There are lots of scientific papers on DLB but the paper we cited above by McKeith *et al.* (2017) provides very good descriptions of the important symptoms.

RESOURCES AND FURTHER READING
DEEP

Dementia Engagement and Empowerment Project is the UK network of dementia voices. DEEP consists of around 80 groups of people with dementia across the UK.

www.dementiavoices.org.uk

Dementia guide
DEMENTIA, SOCIAL SERVICES AND THE NHS

www.nhs.uk/conditions/dementia/social-services-and-the-nhs

Carer's assessment

The carer's assessment is a process where your local authority or local council social services assess your individual needs as a carer.

www.dementiauk.org/get-support/legal-and-financial-information/the-carers-assessment

Lewy Body Society

www.lewybody.org

A GUIDE TO LEWY BODY DEMENTIA

www.lewybody.org/download/a-guide-to-lewy-body-dementia-2021-edition/?wpdmdl=5427&refresh=614c65672edd81632396647

UNDERSTANDING LEWY BODY DEMENTIA

www.lewybody.org/wp-content/uploads/2021/05/Understanding-Lewy-body-dementia.pdf

MANAGING HALLUCINATIONS AND CHANGES IN VISUAL PERCEPTION IN LEWY BODY DEMENTIA

www.lewybody.org/download/managinghallucinations/?wpdmdl=28648&refresh=614c6567335b61632396647

DIAMOND-Lewy

A programme of research that promotes an assessment and management tool throughout the NHS, with subsequent wide impact in terms of improving patient care for those with Lewy body dementia.

https://research.ncl.ac.uk/diamondlewy

CHAPTER 10

'He's run away with another woman'

FALSE BELIEFS AND DELUSIONS

Jane Hall (pseudonym)

It all started when Dad died. Mum didn't believe he was dead and insisted that he had run away with another woman, a nearby neighbour. Whenever she saw this woman standing outside the car, she would shout, 'Run her over!' We would try to prove that Dad was dead by showing Mum the funeral order of service and reminding her of the presence of people known to us, and her, at the funeral. Although this would work short-term, it would eventually revert back to her belief that Dad had run away with the neighbour.

Next came the belief that she was being robbed. Mum would be adamant that someone was entering the house and taking jewellery and money. We would find the money and her rings behind cushions, in pockets, under mats and in various places hidden around the house. Mum would say she hadn't put it there and it must have been the thieves who had hidden it so they could return later to collect it. She would tell us elaborate stories of how she would wake up and find the thieves, who would then run away, and the police would come to arrest them, which was all untrue.

Mum began to believe her house, which she had lived in for the past 25 years, was in fact a hotel and she wanted to 'go back home' to be with her mother and sisters. She would get packed and wait with her hat, coat and cases ready when I got there to make her evening meal, and it would take a long time to convince her to stay in her own home.

Over the many months Mum held these false beliefs, I tried to convince her to go to the GP or to arrange for the GP to come to visit her at home, but she steadfastly refused and would become suspicious and distressed, so I stopped trying to persuade her to do so and tried to muddle through as best I could.

SPECIALIST COMMENTARY

Dr Malsha Gunathilake, MTI Trainee in Psychiatry (International Training Fellow), Havering Older Adults Mental Health and Memory Service, NELFT, and **Dr Janet Carter**, Associate Professor, Division of Psychiatry UCL, Consultant Old Age Psychiatrist Havering Older Adults Mental Health and Memory Service, NELFT

What are false beliefs and delusions?
FALSE BELIEFS

Everyone has their own beliefs regarding the world, people and events around them. Usually, these beliefs are based on our experience, knowledge and socio-cultural background, and they influence how we view the world. False beliefs are common to us all. For example, we may jump to the conclusion that a 'lost' wallet has been stolen. However, the ability to recognise and remember allows us to consider other possibilities such as whether the wallet is forgotten and still at home – a belief that we can then 'reality-check' when the wallet is found.

The limitations caused by cognitive impairment mean that people with dementia cannot check with reality and correct or moderate their beliefs in this way. Consequently, these false beliefs can become prominent and persist despite evidence to the contrary (Ballard *et al.* 1995).

DELUSIONS

Delusions are firmly held false beliefs that are not based on reality. However, they are real and true to the person with dementia and cannot be changed by challenging or reasoning. In the example above, Jane's mother is convinced that her jewellery and money have been stolen by thieves. When the family finds them hidden around the house later, she makes sense of this different reality by believing that the thieves have hidden them, simply to collect them later. She does not accept that they are not stolen and that she has misplaced them or hidden them to keep them safe.

Nearly one-third of people with dementia experience delusions. The prevalence of delusions varies in different types of dementias:

- dementia with Lewy bodies (DLB): 55–75 per cent

- dementia in Parkinson's disease: 32–63 per cent

- Alzheimer's disease: 11–17 per cent

- vascular dementia: 5–14 per cent

- frontotemporal dementia: 1.2–13 per cent.

The commonest types of delusions found in people with dementia are:

- Delusions of reference (22%) – a belief that others are talking about them or that the actions of others have special reference to them. For example, someone may believe that their husband and children are talking about them each time they see them talking with each other.

- Delusions of theft or possessions being hidden (22%) – a belief that others are stealing or hiding their belongings.

- Delusions of strangers in the house (21%) – a belief that unknown people are inside or occupying the house.

- Delusions of persecution (17%) – a belief that others are trying to harm, kill or poison them.

- Delusions of infidelity – a belief that the partner is unfaithful and is having other relationships without any sound evidence (as in the example above).

- Delusions of misidentification – a belief that a known person has been replaced by an imposter even though their appearance is the same, or a belief that a known person changes their appearance or comes in different disguises to harm them.

Delusions in dementia cause distress to the individual and may lead to irritability, agitation and aggression towards others. The individual may act on their beliefs – for example, by calling the police to report a theft or intruders in their home. This significantly increases the burden for those caring and supporting, especially if the false beliefs are directed at them. Unlike in other mental illness such as schizophrenia, delusions in dementia are generally not long-lasting, tending to fluctuate and change in theme and content as in the example above.

Why do delusions occur in dementia?

Progressive degenerative changes take place in the brain in dementia: loss of neurons, brain circuit changes and changes in neurotransmitters including dopamine, serotonin and glutamate. These changes reduce the ability of the brain to 'process' incoming information correctly. The occurrence of delusions can be explained biologically by these neurological processes.

There are other causes that can lead to the origin of false beliefs and delusions. Memory loss about recent events, conversations and experiences can result in subsequent attempts to 'fill the gap' with false details. Lack of recognition may lead to false beliefs about surroundings, resulting in a desire to 'go home' to a remembered familiar place such as a childhood home. Loss of more recent memories with retention of only older remote memories as the illness progresses may also impact recognition of current places and people. In the above example, Jane's mother no longer recognises her own home, substituting the false but plausible belief that she must be in a hotel. Similarly, changes in routine, environment and regular caregivers, and poor hearing and vision can all contribute to misinterpretation of events and surroundings.

Sudden onset of delusions or rapid worsening of confusion with or without hallucinations in a person with dementia may indicate onset of delirium (see Chapter 8) and warrant further immediate investigation.

A helpful approach: the 3 Rs – reassure, respond and refocus

If a delusion does not cause significant problems to the person with dementia or to others, 'letting it lie' is a good approach. Sensitively responding to the real emotion evoked by the delusion – for example, fear, sadness, loneliness, anger – and offering explanations and reassurance without challenging the belief can be helpful. In Jane's situation, instead of reminding her mother that her husband is dead and there is no family home to go to, an approach might be to ask about childhood memories ('Tell me about the house you grew up in'), try to understand why the person believes this is not their home, and to distract them by talking or doing something enjoyable. This approach can be used in the example above where Jane's mother believes her own house to be a hotel.

- Try to identify any causes for the delusion. There may be situational factors – for example, the presence of a new person or a recent change in décor to her environment. Keeping a record of the details of situations (when and where), any events prior to the episode and the resulting beliefs may help to identify precipitating factors which, if changed, would help to reduce delusions.

- Correction of vision and hearing with glasses and hearing aids, respectively, may help in avoiding misinterpretation.

- If someone misplaces the same things repeatedly, having multiples of the same item as backup or establishing an agreed place to keep important items such as keys, may help.

- Distraction and refocusing can help to minimise distress.

Medication

Memory enhancers (donepezil, rivastigmine, memantine) typically used for dementia symptoms can themselves help reduce delusions. If these are not effective and delusions are getting worse and/or are resulting in increased risk to the person with dementia or others around them, adding another medication called an antipsychotic medication can be justified. This will only be considered by a doctor after weighing all risks and benefits because of potential side effects.

The type of medication used depends on the type of dementia and other individual factors. More caution is needed when prescribing antipsychotics to those with dementia with Lewy bodies and dementia in Parkinson's disease than other types of dementia, because of an increased sensitivity to side effects. All antipsychotic medication should be started in a small dose, and it is usually given short-term. If symptoms recur after stopping antipsychotics, a longer trial period may be considered. The common side effects of antipsychotics include tremors, rigidity, weight gain and drowsiness. Antipsychotics are also known to increase the risk of stroke by nearly twofold. Therefore, use of these medications in dementia are considered only as a last resort when other interventions fail or are inadequate.

ADMIRAL NURSE ADVICE

Fiona Chaabane, Consultant Admiral Nurse/ Clinical Nurse Specialist in Younger Onset Dementia and Huntington's Disease, University Hospital Southampton NHS Foundation Trust

False beliefs are not exclusive to dementia and are commonly seen in a range of conditions, each with their own cause and solution. In healthcare, a person who has a high temperature or an infection or who is dehydrated, for example, may experience episodes of false beliefs in which they are convinced that their new (false) beliefs – and all the detail and context surrounding their thoughts – are true and intense, despite reassurance and evidence to the contrary.

At their worst, the person experiencing false beliefs may believe that they are under threat in some way or feel persecuted, that they are at risk or in danger or that something terrible is going to happen. It is hardly surprising therefore that, in this circumstance, the person may appear very distressed and fearful, feel vulnerable and disbelieved, or feel that no one can help them. Anyone observing this, watching the person struggle to make sense of what they believe, may feel helpless themselves and unable to provide comfort. This creates a cycle of distress that encircles both the person affected and the caregiver, often increasing in intensity before the issue can be resolved.

The first step on which to base any approach to a person experiencing false beliefs, for whatever reason, is to understand and appreciate that the person's ideas are only false to the onlooker – the person experiencing them directly will be convinced of their validity and may become further distressed if they feel they are not believed.

The second step is to check the origin of the beliefs, to see if there could be any truth to the distressing thoughts. Cases have been recorded where a person voicing ideas of what appear to be illogical and false beliefs has been entirely correct. This is a particular risk in dementia where it might be easier to attribute what appears to be irrational thinking to cognitive change. A comprehensive account of the history of the beliefs is essential in examination and may provide a clue as to the cause and whether any treatment or management plan is needed.

How our brains make sense of information

In Jane's case, her mother's false beliefs have developed over quite a long period, starting at the time her husband died, and have continued to evolve as her memory and general function declined, affecting her ability to make sense of her environment and relationships. Her false beliefs reflect memory problems, but memory difficulties do not exist in isolation – they are part of a wider system of cognitive function, in how the brain organises its thoughts, how it processes and responds to information, how it makes judgements and links one piece of information to another. These are all functions that are necessary for us to make sense of the information we receive and to put it in order. As these abilities decline, it is likely that the false beliefs change in this context. This is a fault of the brain when filing or storing information – if not stored or 'coded' correctly, the brain will struggle to return to information in the right order at the right time, and some information may be so mis-filed that it cannot be retrieved at all. Unfortunately, in Jane's mother's case, she also lacked any insight into her memory problems and was unable to accept her daughter's reasoning.

An approach that can help

If the person with dementia holds false beliefs and there is no truth to the thoughts, they are incorrect and the person cannot be convinced of the true situation, they are likely to be distressed because their 'truth' is different to what others are telling them. This might then show in a change in mood, an increase in anxiety or agitation, an attempt to leave where they are to 'go home' or persistent efforts to respond to the false beliefs directly. The person may be reluctant to adhere to their usual routine, may resist help or care from others, may not wish to eat or drink, and even sleep may be affected. In the worst-case scenario, they may even become aggressive towards a caregiver for not allowing them to act on their thoughts – for example, by preventing them from leaving or not allowing them to do so something (perhaps perceived as potentially harmful). They may be confused, disorientated or not be sufficiently aware of risk or the stress they are under.

In dementia, this level of anxiety or distress can be hugely disruptive to the brain's need for order and routine and can lead to a worsening of the person's overall mood and general wellbeing. False beliefs therefore present a very real threat to the person's general state of health, and approaches to address them should form an action plan to support the person through these very distressing periods.

Are the false beliefs related to memory loss?

It is important to remember that a person with dementia may lose insight into their needs or deficits quite early on in the illness and may have no awareness at all that they are experiencing cognitive change. From their perspective, a personal item surely must have been moved and consequently lost by someone else, maybe with sinister intent – what else could the explanation be? Perhaps a logical step forward in this circumstance for Jane's mother might be to hide things she wishes to keep safe, but she then forgets where she has placed them and so believes them stolen. Such memory problems can therefore feed a cycle of false beliefs, inappropriate attempts to resolve the problem and a greater level of suspicion over time.

Where these issues relate to the person's short-term memory, together with their difficulties with judgement, it is more likely that the person can be gently distracted from their concerns by someone they feel safe with, trust and with whom they feel they can engage. The person with dementia may respond to reassurance, a calm and unhurried approach, and time to engage that leads to a gentle and positive distraction to another subject or activity. This may need to be repeated many times in a day.

Where there are gaps in a person's recall, the brain tries to manage this by filling in those gaps but doesn't always get this right; the brain needs to be working at its best to be able do this.

Dementia interferes with a lot of brain processes, such as memory storage, which causes increasing difficulties as time goes on and the illness advances. This is not something the person with dementia will have any control over.

Do the false beliefs appear to be intensifying in content and context?

There may be times where no amount of distraction/reassurance or argument can resolve a person's false beliefs, although distraction and reassurance can be very helpful in relieving any associated anxiety or distress. False beliefs can grow in intensity over a short time to engulf the person with dementia and those around them. This can be a very distressing time for all involved but especially for the person with dementia who will not have the ability to resolve their false beliefs by rationally thinking and talking them through, and therefore grounding them in reality.

It is important to seek an assessment by a healthcare professional to rule out any underlying causes, such as an infection or other physical condition that can be remedied with treatment. The person with dementia may be experiencing delirium, in which case treatment of the physical illness will resolve the thought disorder and false beliefs (see Chapter 8).

In some cases, false beliefs can intensify and present a gradually increasing sense of jeopardy to the person with dementia. The person may respond to the threat of a false belief – for example if they believe that their neighbours are trying to harm them, they may take action to protect themselves. There can sometimes be paranoid overtones to some false beliefs, which can be very distressing indeed. As Dr Carter and Dr Gunathilake indicate, there may be instances such as this that require medication (an antipsychotic treatment) to help the brain's connections to stabilise and gradually reduce and stop the false beliefs.

How can an Admiral Nurse support you?

Admiral Nurses are specialists in dementia care and have a wide range of experience and skills in assessing and supporting people with dementia and their families. While each individual case is different in its fabric and features, the difficulties that false beliefs can invoke for family carers are well known to all Admiral Nurses. Through thorough and comprehensive history taking, listening to the person with dementia and their family, understanding the setting and dynamics of the symptoms, the Admiral Nurse will be able to advise on a plan of action to help address the difficulties. This might involve working with other healthcare professionals to ensure the person with dementia receives the clinical help they need. It also means working with those closest to the person with dementia to enable them to respond better to the distress of false beliefs and to help improve the quality of life and experience of the person with dementia.

An Admiral Nurse will 'get it' – will understand and be able to help work towards managing false beliefs safely. Using knowledge and clinical expertise to tailor solutions to the particular needs of the person with dementia and their family members, they are able to address this very distressing aspect of their illness.

REFERENCES

Ballard, C.G., Saad, K., Patel, A., Gahir, M. *et al.* (1995) 'The prevalence and phenomenology of psychotic symptoms in dementia sufferers.' *International Journal of Geriatric Psychiatry 10*, 6, 477–485. doi:10.1002/gps.930100607.

RESOURCES AND FURTHER READING
Dementia UK
FALSE BELIEFS AND DELUSIONS IN DEMENTIA

www.dementiauk.org/get-support/understanding-changes-in-dementia/false-beliefs-and-delusions-in-dementia

COPING WITH DISTRESS

www.dementiauk.org/get-support/understanding-changes-in-dementia/coping-with-distress

CHAPTER 11

'He'd sit in that blessed chair all day, he would'

APATHY IN DEMENTIA

Bridget Culson (pseudonym)

(Bridget has been married to Eric for just over 50 years. They are both in their early 70s.)

It's so hard to get him to do anything these days. He just sits and sits. The TV's on but he's not watching it, could be anything, he couldn't tell you. Drives me bonkers. 'Eric, do you want to do this? Eric, do you want to come out with me?' Either no answer or he just grunts no.

I'll start at the beginning maybe. He was a lovely man, Eric, before all this. Always quite quiet, he was a bit of a little fellow, you know, well quite slim and slight. But always neat and nicely turned out. He preferred to iron his own nice white shirts, didn't really think I did them neat enough. He wasn't great on socialising, but we'd go out, like to the pub or the Irish Club, have a few drinks and that. After a couple of drinks, he might loosen up a bit, start flirting with my girlfriends. I minded at the time, but I'd give anything for him to be able to do that again now. He'd been in the Navy before I knew him and had a lot of very rude jokes that he'd tell back then. He was an electrician – well, they have to be perfectionists, don't they, or else *Boom!* Very neat and careful with his tools, very organised with the business side, too – invoices and tax and all that stuff. I never knew much about money until I had to take it over. He loved fiddling around the house, doing wee jobs, and he had his allotment, too.

When he retired, we were going to travel everywhere and live the high life. Didn't quite work out like that. We did a couple of trips, but Eric found them more like hard work than fun. He seemed worried about losing things or about getting lost. I had to hold his hand a couple of times to calm him down. So we stopped globetrotting and after a little while we weren't really going anywhere. He never suggested doing anything or going anywhere, or there were reasons for not going out. I didn't want to go to the club on my own, so it was either push Eric out the door with me or not go at all. That made for lots of fun, not.

Probably was about then that I started to notice other stuff too. Mainly that he was getting a bit forgetful. I might have to remind him what day it was. He'd start doing something and then seemed to forget what he was trying to do. Like he'd start preparing some woodwork to paint it and then forget. That wasn't like him at all. He was also getting to be less use around the house. I'd have to ask him to do things he'd always done, like putting the bin out. Then I'd have to check that he had. More like, I'd have to remind him again to do it. Quicker to put the thing out myself, in the end. Oh, and he did daft stuff, putting his screwdrivers in the fridge or chucking the bread into the kitchen bin. Gosh, that was irritating, I'd have words, but he didn't seem to react. Not that he ever got into arguments much.

By the time I realised he couldn't go to the shops on his own, I knew something had to be done. Till then, I'd tried to ignore it – you know, 'Perhaps he's just getting old?' But then I'd think, 'Well, Paddy at the club, he's 68 too but he's full of life', and I'd worry that maybe something was wrong with Eric. Sending him to the shops, wow, that was a bit hilarious I suppose, looking back on it. It wasn't at the time. I'd send him off with a list, and he'd buy half the things on it and things we didn't need. He couldn't cope with cash any more as he seemed to think £5 would cover a week's shop. One time he came back with nothing at all. God knows where he'd left the bag; we never found it.

More than anything, though, he seemed to be losing interest in everything. It was a worry, I couldn't interest him in things, couldn't have a bit of chat with him like I used to. If he was to go to the allotment, I'd have to go with him. That wasn't the idea at all – him going to the allotment was my time to put my feet up at home.

Took at least a year to get him to the GP. 'I'm not ill', 'There's nowt wrong with me' – I heard all the excuses. Driving me up the wall as I was getting more and more sure there was something going wrong with him. Cut a long story short, we got referred to the memory clinic. He went to the third appointment they offered; that was only because I threatened to throttle him if he didn't (not that I would have – I love him too much – but maybe you can see how wound up I was getting). Came out with a diagnosis of Alzheimer's disease and some tablets.

That was about two years ago. Since then, it's just got worse. Sits in the same chair – he's wearing it out. He'd sit in that blessed chair all day, he would... TV on, he doesn't change channels or anything, can't tell me what he's been watching. I don't think he follows it. Same with his clothes. He'd wear the same things every day; I have to hide his shirts and trousers sometimes so that I can wash them. They get very mucky as he doesn't care whether he spills food down the front or not. Times he won't even go to the toilet and he's just peed himself in the chair. I'm wise to that, I make him go to the toilet every now and again. And I have to check he's wiped himself when he needs to. Eating? I don't think he'd bother with that either. I have to nag him a bit to come to the table. Sometimes I give up and put it on a tray. Not that he'll eat it unless I sit with him and tell him what to do.

To get him out of the house needs a bit of cunning sometimes. I feel a bit guilty if I'm promising him things, but I have to do whatever I can, don't I? Then if we do go, let's say to the memory café, he sometimes enjoys it. Sometimes not, he'll just sit there; other times, suddenly he's quite bright and a bit chatty. You never can tell. Or if the grandchildren come – most times he can't even remember their names – but sometimes he lights up for a bit – it's lovely to see. Although then he gets tired and he's had enough.

Dear me, it's a struggle. I get that tired, I may just collapse in a heap. What happens then? Goodness knows, I don't like to think about it. I just plod on, nag nag, try to do my best, keep trying to find that little spark that gets him going.

SPECIALIST COMMENTARY

Professor Tom Dening, Professor of Dementia Research, and **Dr Malarvizhi Babu Sandilyan**, Consultant in Old Age Psychiatry

What is apathy?

Apathy describes several things, including a mental state of not caring or being indifferent to things, a lack of motivation and inability to initiate activity, and the accompanying behaviour where someone appears to lack interest or energy and may also seem unwilling to do anything. In slightly more scientific language, apathy has cognitive, emotional and behavioural components. That is to say, it affects the way people think (e.g. not being bothered about anything or motivated to do anything), how they feel (often indifferent) and how they behave (not doing very much unless prodded to do so).

Apathy is one of the commonest features of dementia, and it occurs to some degree in between 50 and 75 per cent of people with the condition (Selbæk, Engedal and Bergh 2013). As in Eric's case, it may start quite early in the course of dementia, so that the person seems to lose interest in things they used to enjoy such as hobbies and pastimes, or does not want social contact.

Eric's apathy

One of the first signs of Eric's dementia was that he stopped wanting to travel or even go out to the club. He seemed to lose interest in doing jobs around the house. In part, this was probably due to other problems arising from the dementia – for example, he was forgetting what he'd already done and putting his tools away in the wrong places, which would have been due to memory loss. But he also became less motivated to start doing anything, and that is characteristic of apathy. At first, though, it can be difficult to tell if a person is starting to slow down, and it is often simply ascribed to their age. It is usually only when other symptoms of dementia, such as forgetfulness, start to become troublesome that the significance of the apathy is realised. Bridget only started to worry about the apathy when other things went wrong, too.

As dementia progresses, so too does apathy. Eric became less interested in conversation – again, that may be partly due to other difficulties, not just the apathy. For example, if Eric has Alzheimer's disease, he may also be having trouble finding the right words for things (aphasia) and that can make it so difficult to hold a conversation that the other person eventually simply gives up trying. This, of course, fits alongside the apathy, which also reduces their motivation to communicate. Bridget also tells us about Eric's reluctance to go to the allotment or to attend the hospital clinic.

At the time of Bridget's story, Eric's dementia has progressed further and now it's probably the apathy that is the main problem. Eric sits all day in the same chair. He doesn't change his clothes or wash unless strongly encouraged to do so. He shows no interest in anything around him. To get him out of the house requires a major effort from Bridget. Not surprisingly, she finds all this extremely frustrating. She is not alone. Apathy is certainly one of the most difficult features of dementia for family carers and causes high levels of stress and a sense of burden for them, as we see in Bridget's case.

However, despite all the difficulty and frustration, there are some brighter moments. For example, if the grandchildren visit or on the rare occasions that Bridget can get Eric to attend a social group, then suddenly he will brighten up and show some of his old self. Family carers will often work very hard to achieve this sort of moment because, even if it is brief, it provides a reminder that the person with dementia is still a real person, not just an empty shell.

What causes apathy?

Apathy is associated with brain disease such as dementia and is partly due to changes in certain areas of the brain. The brain region behind the forehead, the frontal lobes, controls our ability to plan, focus and maintain motivation. The frontal lobes have rich connections with other areas of the brain, forming a series of neuronal circuits that are responsible for 'goal-directed behaviour' – that is, our ability to focus on a task and respond appropriately.

When the frontal lobes and its connections are affected by dementia, people tend to become passive and less motivated, although sometimes they can also become disinhibited and behave in an over-familiar or inappropriate way. Similarly, people who develop vascular dementia due to strokes in the frontal region of their brain are more likely to develop apathy. Apathy is often associated with Alzheimer's disease in people who have reduced activity in the frontal and mid-brain regions and changes in levels of certain neurochemicals, such as acetylcholine and dopamine.

However, it is important to think about other factors, besides just brain disease, that may contribute to apathy in dementia. It is clear from Eric's story that he is not equally apathetic all the time, so there must be other factors at work, which may be related to his own mental state but also to the environment around him.

Apathy is also closely related to depression. Indeed, it is a common symptom of depression especially if the depression is moderate or severe. It is quite common to see people with depression losing interest in work or activities, and at times they may neglect their appearance or other aspects of self-care. However, apathy and depression are separate entities since either can occur without the other. It's important in assessing a patient with dementia, like Eric, to check whether they might be depressed as well as having apathy, in which case prescribing an antidepressant may be helpful.

Why apathy matters

Apathy is often associated with reduced quality of life in people affected with dementia. Apathy tends to become more marked as the dementia progresses. People with apathy and dementia show reduced independence in activities of daily living, poor outcomes with rehabilitation, and higher mortality.

As discussed previously, apathy often overlaps with depressive symptoms, with patients spiralling into a cycle of lethargy and lack of motivation or effort. Apathy can be very frustrating to live with, especially when family carers misunderstand the apathy as being merely lazy or wilful, rather than a result of the dementia. We can clearly see this from Bridget's experience. Along with carer burden, there is also an economic burden, as higher rates of apathy are associated with increased rates of admission to a care setting.

The experience of having apathy

We have heard from Bridget about the experience of being the carer for a person with dementia who has a profound degree of apathy. But what about Eric? How does the world seem to him? For example, does he even realise that there's a problem?

Not surprisingly, this is not an easy area to research since a person with dementia and apathy may not only lack motivation to respond but may also struggle to find words to describe their experiences. Some themes that emerge from research (Baber *et al.* 2021; Chang *et al.* 2021) into patient and carer experience are a sense of losing themselves, feeling like a burden, and the invisible obstacles against which they struggle to try to keep in contact with others. Family carers also describe negative emotions, such as guilt and frustration, and positive sentiments, such as wanting to reignite their partners' 'spark' if they can. People with apathy also describe things that keep them going, which include their desire to be helpful and to stay involved, the importance of keeping a routine and retaining their usual habits as much as possible.

It is easy to see Bridget's experiences reflected in the findings from this research, since she describes being irritated, frustrated and tired. She uses cunning in order to get Eric to do what she needs him to. And she is constantly looking for ways in which he can be stimulated and show a bit of his old self. As to Eric's experience, we can only surmise, but it seems plausible that he realises he can't do things that he used to do easily. He will doubtless realise that he needs his wife to help him a lot, which may make him feel a burden to her. Furthermore, he is probably trying to do his best, wanting to be helpful and do the right thing, but struggling against invisible obstacles. Maybe this is a bit like wading through quicksand and at the same time being unable to call for help.

What can we do about apathy?

Various pharmacological treatments have been proposed for treating apathy in dementia, although none is especially effective. These include the drugs called acetylcholinesterase inhibitors (donepezil, rivastigmine and galantamine), which are used to treat the cognitive symptoms of Alzheimer's disease and may also be beneficial in treating non-cognitive symptoms too, such as depression, anxiety and apathy. However, despite some initially promising results, data combined from several studies show no significant effects. Our own clinical experience suggests that, for some patients at least, acetylcholinesterase inhibitors do sometimes have quite a marked alerting effect on patients, so that they are able to focus their attention better and, for example, make more effort to participate in conversations. There is little evidence that any other drugs help to improve apathy, except perhaps the stimulant drug methylphenidate.

Non-pharmacological approaches are therefore of great importance and are the mainstay for helping people with apathy and their family carers. These include a whole range of activities, which our Admiral Nurse colleague will discuss.

When we think closely about the experiences of people like Eric and Bridget, maybe what would be helpful is greater recognition of apathy and how important it is as a feature of dementia. If they both had a better explanation of the symptom, then perhaps Bridget would be less inclined to think that Eric is being wilful. She might understand better just how difficult it is for him and how much he is in fact struggling to help, even though there is no visible sign of this. Similarly, it may have helped Eric to know more about apathy much earlier in the course of his dementia, so that they could both have worked harder at trying to maintain his routine and his favourite activities.

What recent research tells us is that apathy is a vitally important part of dementia. We have tended to emphasise the importance of memory, partly because it is easier to describe and easier to measure, but we should pay much more attention to apathy. There should be better information about it for professionals and for the public. Maybe we should start running apathy cafés, too?

ADMIRAL NURSE ADVICE

Lucy Chamberlain, Admiral Nurse, Royal British Legion

How it can feel to care for someone with apathy

First of all, it's important to know that this is a really common feature of dementia, and it can often be a significant cause of frustration for family carers – it's a real thing, and it's OK to get a bit fed up sometimes!

It can seem as if the person with dementia has 'given up' or lost the ability or confidence to perform tasks, and it can be really upsetting when the person seems totally disinterested in their loved ones or their news. In some cases, people with dementia may even retreat to their bed and seem to spend large portions of the day and night 'just lying there awake'. Family carers have described it as like 'living with a ghost' and say they feel guilty about being frustrated, even becoming angry, and feeling that the person with dementia is behaving like this deliberately. Many family carers feel a sense of burden or responsibility in that they feel they should be doing more to engage with the person with dementia to give them a better quality of life, or that the apathy may be down to something they are not doing or not doing well enough.

Once we can explain to family carers the reasons why the person with dementia has become affected by apathy, as we see in Bridget and Eric's case, this can not only remove some of the guilt but also help them to understand that there are a few things we can try to help.

As Professor Dening and Dr Sandilyan explain, a prescription of antidepressants and/or anticholinesterase inhibitors (the dementia medications) may be worth trying. However, it is important to first rule out any other causes for the person with dementia seeming unwilling to do things – for example, pain that is only eased when sitting or lying still, or eyesight problems meaning they are frightened to move about.

Routines and personal hygiene

Routines are very helpful for all of us, and even more so for busy family carers where the person with dementia is experiencing apathy. A routine may have several benefits, such as helping to ensure important things get done, and could include regularly helping the person with dementia with personal care, such as cleaning of teeth and changing clothes. Removing soiled clothing to the wash basket as soon as it is taken off and laying out the next day's clean clothes can be helpful and avoids the effort it may take for the person with dementia to choose clothing on a day-to-day basis. Perhaps an evening bathing routine, while helping with hygiene and changing clothes, may have been something the person previously enjoyed. Setting the environment to be pleasurable and soothing – a pleasant-smelling bath oil, warm room, calm music, low lighting and so forth – will make it more appealing and encourage their engagement.

The very nature of a routine is that it brings predictability to one's life, which can have a reassuring effect on the person with dementia by allowing them a sense of safety in this strange new world and enabling them to feel a connection with their previous habits and preferences. People with dementia may often return to behaviours from many years ago, so knowing what these were will help you to plan successful routines. For example, some family carers find that the person with dementia no longer enjoys taking a shower, but is more accepting of a bath, perhaps as they may have been used to bathing before showers became more common. Other things relating to personal hygiene might be reverting back to a particular time of day they used to prefer to wash, or their electric toothbrush may now feel unfamiliar, so going back to a traditional-style brush may help. Sometimes even a new brand of toothpaste tasting too strong may cause disengagement with teeth cleaning. It is OK to experiment to try to find the components of a routine that achieve the best results – this sort of thing can be influenced by previous preferences or lifestyle or may even be found by trial and error.

A routine may also help in preventing problems, for example, with continence. Apathy may mean people do not recognise the need to go to the toilet, or be slow to react to the feeling, and so regularly prompting or taking someone to the toilet may reduce the likelihood of accidents, as Bridget found with Eric. Such routines may take the pressure off both of you; the person with dementia gets the help they need, and the carer doesn't have to 'think of everything' as it is part of their daily routine.

Food and apathy

As Bridget found with Eric, it may be difficult to motivate some-one with apathy to eat. Again, it's worth making sure there are no underlying problems – for example, a sore or dry mouth is worth checking out with the dentist. Problems with swallowing or a fear of choking – common symptoms in dementia – may be a reason for Eric's reluctance to eat, so it is worth seeking the advice of your GP. Oral thrush can be quite a common problem with people who are apathetic, eating little and/or on medication. This not only makes the mouth sore but can reduce the sense of taste. It is easily treated with medication from the GP.

Providing cues and sticking to habits can be helpful – if they see the table laid and people sitting eating together, this may prompt the person with dementia to recognise it is a meal time. If they used to have their main meal at lunchtime many years ago, this may be a better time now, rather than in the evening. Providing food they really enjoy, even if there is quite a bit of repetition in their diet, is better than eating very little, and perhaps trying foods with an evocative or tempting smell will also encourage eating. If people are unable to settle at the table, eating from a tray, as Bridget did, is ideal, or even providing small, bite-sized finger foods left out nearby so the person with dementia can pick them up when they see them or feel the need to eat.

Activities for people with dementia who experience apathy

People with dementia can be overwhelmed by too much choice or be unable to decide between options, which can be particularly problematic for a person experiencing apathy. Reducing options and making some activities automatic may be beneficial.

If people have lost the ability to initiate or sequence activities for themselves, we can help by starting an activity with them or modelling activities together. This is where dementia care can become personalised to the needs of an individual. As we see in Eric's case, he seemed to perk up more in social and family situations, so where the lead or impetus is taken by someone else, these are more likely to be successful for him. Trying out activities that are more meaningful for the person with dementia and easier to manage are more likely to be successful.

Research has shown that activities that stimulate multiple senses, such as cooking, music, pet therapy and exercise, are all beneficial where a person with dementia experiences apathy, as are structured exercise sessions, such as walking or other forms of exercise. Many peer support groups offer walking or group exercise activities. Individualised cognitive training, intended to stimulate the brain's functioning, such as thinking, speech and memory, based on the person's interests, can impact upon apathy. Other activities that have been found useful for some family carers may include:

- Music, in the form of a personalised playlist for the person with dementia.

- An activity could be as simple as just having paper and a basic paint box or chunky crayons, and letting the person explore the paper. There are dedicated art therapists at some dementia care venues.

- Multisensory stimulation is where the senses – hearing, seeing, smelling, tasting and touch – are stimulated. For example, some people with dementia gain comfort from feeling different textures, such as a piece of cloth with buttons and zips, that they can explore with their hands. Walking through a garden with scented flowers can help stimulate the sense of smell.

- Simulated presence using taped conversations, such as a recording of voices from family for whom visiting is difficult, was very useful during COVID-19.

Overall, maintaining good social relationships and engaging in interpersonal interactions are beneficial for people affected by apathy. Various resources are available that can be used by family carers to engage the person based on their interests, which include kits and apps for cognitive stimulation. Local libraries are worth checking out as they loan dementia-friendly memory bags, puzzles and games, as well as books that might spark conversations about the local area or previous hobbies or jobs.

All of this can be quite emotionally and physically labour-intensive for family carers, so it is equally important that you ensure some rest time for you, too – whether that's meeting friends, reading a book or joining your own exercise class. So reach out for help from family, friends or local services, such as day care or respite, to help you with this.

REFERENCES

Baber, W., Chang, C.Y.M., Yates, J. and Dening, T. (2021) 'The experience of apathy in dementia: A qualitative study.' *International Journal of Environmental Research and Public Health 18*, 6, 3325. doi:10.3390/ijerph18063325.

Chang, C.Y.M., Baber, W., Dening T. and Yates, J. (2021) '"He just doesn't want to get out of the chair and do it": The impact of apathy in people with dementia on their carers.' *International Journal of Environmental Research and Public Health 18*, 12, 6317. doi:10.3390/ijerph18126317.

Selbæk, G., Engedal, K. and Bergh, S. (2013) 'The prevalence and course of neuropsychiatric symptoms in nursing home patients with dementia: A systematic review.' *Journal of American Medical Directors Association 14*, 3, 161–169. doi:10.1016/j.jamda.2012.09.027.

RESOURCES AND FURTHER READING
Dementia UK
MEANINGFUL ACTIVITIES PART FIVE: KEEPING THE
MIND FIT DURING PERIODS OF ISOLATION

www.dementiauk.org/cognitive-stimulation

Social Care Institute for Excellence (SCIE)
ACTIVITY RESOURCES AND APPROACHES FOR DEMENTIA

www.scie.org.uk/dementia/living-with-dementia/keeping-active/activity-resources.asp?gclid=EAIaIQobChMIp8GVtP2F8wIVGeDtCh3ZhwDgEAAYAyAAEgIJXPD_BwE

Playlist for Life
PERSONAL MUSIC FOR DEMENTIA

www.playlistforlife.org.uk

MUSIC FOR MY MIND

https://musicformymind.com

Dementia Adventure
Helping people with dementia and their families to get outdoors and connect with nature, themselves and their communities.

https://dementiaadventure.co.uk

CHAPTER 12

'Where is your father?'

BEREAVEMENT AND DEMENTIA

Surinder Bangar

My mother is 83. She was diagnosed with Alzheimer's disease in April 2014 and was supported by my father until his death in May 2020 from COVID-19. What follows is an account of what happened as we cared for my mother in the months that followed. My parents and their three eldest children (myself included) were all born in India. My father came to the UK in 1964. My mother, together with the three eldest children, joined him in 1966. We are Punjabi Sikhs. In our home, we usually refer to my mother as Bibi and I'll sometimes use this term in the text. After my father's death, our initial focus was upon Bibi. She too had contracted COVID-19 but was slowly recovering, although this was intertwined with the impact of bereavement. Thankfully, Bibi recovered from COVID-19 and after three weeks we were able to see signs of improving physical health.

As a family, we were ill-equipped to understand the impact of bereavement with Alzheimer's disease and there was no information provided to us about this. My mother had returned to the hospital to see my father, although, sadly, by the time she arrived with my siblings, my father had passed away. It was heart-wrenching to witness my mother speaking with my father and unable in that moment to understand why he wasn't talking to her. The next few days became a blur for us all with relatives and family friends paying their respects. These were carried out at a distance and the traditional mourning rituals were not possible because of COVID-19. Comfort for my mother in the form of hugs and being together with our wider family was not possible.

Bibi would continuously ask where our father was. When we explained that he'd passed away, the intensity of her grief would repeat over and over. She would be flailing and in despair. This cycle would continue through the night. To enable my mother to rest and recover from her own COVID-19 illness, initially we occasionally said that our father was at the hospital. This seemed to be something that she would accept in those moments. I was unsure how a person with Alzheimer's processes bereavement or whether it is possible to go through the stages of grief when there are changes taking place in the brain.

It felt as though we were needing to work things out day by day with my mother. There was no blueprint for any of us. At times, it felt as though there was nothing we could do to stop the intensity of the cycles of ongoing grief for my mother. It felt as though, each time, she experienced it anew with overwhelming grief and shock. As she was unable to remember what had happened, she would ask, 'Where is your father?' She knew there was something that she should know, yet she seemed unable to access this information. Responses to this would prompt sobbing and a flurry of questions which repeated over and over as she understandably struggled with the impact of this news. Bibi would repeat, 'He's dead, he's dead? ... I don't believe this... what happened? ... Take me to see him.' Another impact on Bibi was that it seemed to generate fears about what would happen to her: 'No, I can't be on my own, I've never lived alone... Why hasn't he taken me with him? ... Why would god do this?'

My mother would nod when I'd say, 'He had a chest infection.' She would nod and say, 'Yes, he used to get chest infections.' She would say, 'Why can't I remember this, I'm going mental.'

I would respond by saying, 'You were also unwell, you also had an infection, and shock also takes place.' My responses with Bibi usually involved gently responding to her questions, caressing her forehead when she was lying down, keeping a hand on her arm, shoulders, hugging her – just making sure that she had some physical touch to reassure her. Although I felt inadequate in responding to the enormity of what my mother was going through, it felt important to respond in ways that would make sense for her and to talk in Punjabi to help her feel comfortable and to make things easier for her.

My mother became agitated when she asked to see him, to see his body, and culturally this felt important to her. I would say, 'You were at the hospital, you were able to see him, you talked with him, he held your hands' (and at this point I would clasp her hands in mine). Over time, she would repeat this when describing this to herself. 'Yes, he held my hands, I remember.' Whether she remembered or not, it was an important part of feeling that she was with him, that she hadn't let him down and that he did what he was able with her to acknowledge their lives together.

Talking about being in shock and other conversations began to provide a way for Bibi to describe what happened when other people close to her passed away. She started to talk about our Baba (grandad) and she spoke of how he'd passed away unexpectedly: 'We'd just been to see him at the hospital and the next day he was dead.'

There have been some cycles of intense grief since those early days, although they are not as prolonged. Every day that I have been with my mother, in the early hours of the morning, she starts each day grieving for her husband. In looking for information that might help me, I read some accounts of family carers' experiences of looking after loved ones with dementia, but these didn't shed much light on this area. I appreciate that there is no fixed template, and that as my mother's Alzheimer's inevitably progresses, there may be further changes to how she makes sense of people around her, and she may refer to my father as though he is still alive.

In my workplace, I can access bereavement support, and my GP practice can also offer me counselling; however, for my mother living with Alzheimer's, there doesn't seem to be the same access to services or information provided. I feel that more information and support about Alzheimer's and bereavement would be helpful, particularly culturally specific guidance.

SPECIALIST COMMENTARY

Dr E. Joanna Alexjuk, Lecturer, Counselling, Psychotherapy and Applied Social Science, University of Edinburgh

Truth-telling or non-truth-telling: a person-centred approach to supporting a bereaved person with dementia

Caring for someone with dementia has been described as feeling like a 36-hour day (Mace and Rabins 2021). This includes not only aspects of physical support but also providing emotional support, which may involve having to respond to repetitive questions from the family member with dementia, while also negotiating an appropriate approach to limit further distress. However, Surinder's experience offers an additional and challenging factor in relation to her role as a family caregiver. Her extremely personal and sensitive account tells us of her supportive care to her mother, Bibi, who has dementia, as well as the challenge of both her parents contracting COVID-19, and subsequently, the emotional difficulties of then experiencing not only the death of her father, who was Bibi's main carer, but also her own grief and loss of her father.

Surinder's narrative emphasises an intensified and complex situation that both she and other family members faced in supporting Bibi, and each other, through bereavement. This was during a time when the constraints of social distancing measures for the pandemic meant family members were unable to offer physical comfort and undertake the normative traditions and rituals of mourning. There is limited guidance or, as Surinder points out, no definitive 'blueprint' for family carers as to how they can appropriately communicate the loss of a family member to the person with dementia. Nonetheless, Surinder repeatedly conveyed the loss of her father in a loving and caring manner, which included aspects of truth-telling and justifiable non-truth-telling to address Bibi's cyclical responses of yearning, sadness and overwhelming grief in relation to the loss of her husband.

Different realities and beliefs

People with dementia can often experience a different reality and a set of beliefs to those around them (Mental Health Foundation 2016).

This can vary in people with dementia and is dependent on the type of dementia diagnosed, but can also become more frequent and persistent as their condition progresses. These experiences often cause significant distress for them and for the people supporting them. It is especially challenging when the person with dementia is told of the death of someone who was close to them, and may not be able to understand or retain the information. However, the way in which a person with dementia responds is unique to each individual (Duffy and Ballentine 2020), and their process of mourning may differ, with some researchers describing people with dementia as not possessing a 'conventional' ability to interpret and work through their grief and to come to terms with their loss (Watanabe and Suwa 2017).

Truth-telling

The concept of 'truth' is difficult to define, but 'truth-telling' is extremely important and relates to the way in which most people wish to give and receive information. Conveying the truth and supporting a person with dementia, especially within the context of bereavement, is extremely difficult. There may be fluctuating periods of awareness where the person is fully aware of their loss, only for them to become confused and believing the deceased person is still alive. This may result in them searching for them and asking questions of their whereabouts. This can become a cyclical occurrence where the person with dementia and family members find themselves in a repetitive and distressing situation.

Non-truth-telling and therapeutic lies

In contrast, the application of non-truth-telling – sometimes referred to as therapeutic lying – as an attempt to address the needs of the person with dementia is considered to be complex and controversial but often used and seen as an acceptable communication strategy, specifically in addressing emotive issues where repetitive correction may cause further distress to the person with dementia. However, employing a non-truth response within a situation like the one Surinder is experiencing can be challenging with a constant feeling that they may be doing something wrong. For family carers, it is important to consider the concept and application of untruths within a broader context of person-centred and an event-specific approach of communication.

Applying a person-centred response

Theories relating to person-centred care are neither new nor revolutionary. Its origins go back more than 50 years and help us in the application of an active and non-judgemental approach of listening. Person-centred theory in relation to dementia care was further developed by Tom Kitwood in the 1980s, in which he advocated that 'the person still comes first', emphasising the importance of effective communication and relationships. As in Bibi's case, she was aware that something was not quite right, described as a generalised feeling of 'wrong being' (Duffy and Ballentine 2020). This led Bibi to express her sense of 'wrong being' of grief in the form of agitation, restlessness and confusing the recent loss with one experienced previously.

Family carers need to address repetitive questions in a calm and clear manner, while avoiding euphemisms such as 'passed away' or 'at peace now'. If possible, one family member should take the lead on this and allow Bibi plenty of time within a quiet and calm environment, as Surinder did so well. However, questions may be asked at different times of the day or night when other family members or caregivers are there, so a collective response should be agreed upon for consistency – for example, when the deceased person would be leaving or returning home from work, or at family events, those 'special times' that had previously been shared and were an important part of their relationship. However, it is important to acknowledge that the question as to where the deceased person is might simply mean they want to talk about them, as indeed we all do in coming to terms with the loss of a loved one, so keeping sentences short and offering physical touch is important.

ADMIRAL NURSE ADVICE

Chris O'Connor, Admiral Nurse, Sussex and Surrey Healthcare, and **Deborah Hutchinson**, Admiral Nurse, DUK Helpline

Grief is a normal response to loss

As Surinder comments, there is no universal template to fit all people with dementia to support their individual experiences of grief. People with dementia still feel grief when someone close dies, either imme-diately after the death or over time or in waves, very much like we all do as human beings. Also, it is not uncommon for family members to feel they should protect the person from experiencing distress and try to avoid talking about the death. However, grief is part of a normal emotional response to loss and death. Surindar instinctively realised this, and, though both difficult and painful for her, she enabled her mother to feel and acknowledge her grief as it came in waves to her conscious mind and was there to support her through this.

Allowing her mother to grieve and cry was important as it not only enabled Bibi to express her emotions but also validated her emotional response to her husband's death and meant she did not bottle this up. Crying helps our body to release stress hormones, such as cortisol, which can cause physical and emotional stress if we allow it to build up in our bodies. Similarly, another benefit of crying at such times is that it stimulates our body's production of endorphins. An endorphin is another hormone produced by our body to ease pain and make us feel calmer and happier. Endorphins are sometimes called 'natural pain killers', since that's the way they act in the body. Things like stress and exercise can stimulate the release of endorphins.

Sharing news of a death with someone with dementia
There are some things you can do to help when breaking the news to a person with dementia that someone close to them has died:

- Agree on a consistent approach across family members.

- When breaking bad news, such as a death, to someone with dementia, it is important for family members to consider their stage of dementia and their relationship to the deceased. If the person with dementia was not often in contact with the individual who has died, it may be appropriate not to share the news. If it is someone more meaningful, they may already sense that something is wrong, so gauge this and respond to both their verbal and non-verbal forms of communication. Use short, simple sentences and clear language – for example, say the person has 'died' instead of using euphemisms like 'passed away'.

- Choose a time when the individual is well rested. Morning tends to be a good time for activities and delivering important information.

- Share the news as soon as possible, especially if the person's absence is causing agitation.

What if they forget after I have told them?

Sometimes the person with dementia may forget the death has occurred and will need to be told a second or third time. It is important that they have a chance to grieve in their own way to help emotional acceptance and physical yearning. However, as in Surinder's case, other family members may also be struggling with their own grief and may feel it is upsetting to relive the grief with the person with dementia. Highly emotional events in daily life can be preserved in memory, and such memory is generally referred to as emotional memory (Okada and Matsuo 2012). Although the person with dementia may forget the details or facts of the death, the emotional impact may remain in their memory for some time. Sometimes allowing the person to talk about the deceased person may help with the recall of their death. However, if the person with dementia needs to be told several times and is just not retaining this information, it is OK to stop repeating and breaking the bad news and consider other strategies.

If they ask for the deceased person, as does Bibi – 'Where is your father?' – perhaps try alternative responses, such as they are resting or have gone to visit someone. Everyone grieves differently and it may be the case, as with Surinder, that the family carer may need to support the person with dementia through the intense feelings of grief for some time.

Involve the person with dementia in any funeral or commemoration arrangements

If the person with dementia can and wants to, they should be given the opportunity to help plan the funeral or ceremony for the deceased person. Funerals are a significant life event, and although the person with dementia may forget day-to-day activities, this type of event tends to be one that they will recall. This will allow them to reminisce and be involved in preparatory activities, such as choosing significant photographs for the order of service, music to be sung or played, and memories of that person's life for a eulogy. As with Surinder's mother, it may also prompt discussion about family or cultural traditions used to say goodbye to someone who has died. These can then be used as a tool after the funeral also to aid talking about the person and supporting any grief reaction in the person with dementia.

Keeping photographs of the person on display in their home, copies of the order of service, favourite flowers and pieces of music can all aid positive recollections of the deceased for the person with dementia. If the person with dementia is unable to retain that the person has died, you can still speak about them in the past tense through recollecting and sharing memories. It is important to consider the mood of the person with dementia at such times; if they seem agitated or upset, offer comfort and modify the way you share and discuss the mementos.

Taking care of yourself

Supporting the person with dementia through their grief can often result in the carer feeling that they don't get time to grieve themselves. There may be a tendency to hide emotions from the person with dementia, including crying, to maintain their emotional equilibrium. The best way to support a person with dementia who may be grieving is to make sure you are taking care of yourself through your own grieving process. To be able to effectively support the person with dementia means you have to first be in the best place yourself. There are certain activities you can use to help you to grieve in a managed way. For example, use a particular piece of music that reminds you of the deceased person and allows yourself to think of them while it plays. Keep a grief journal or diary to share your thoughts and feelings. The CRUSE bereavement support organisation has many ideas about ways to support yourself through the grieving process; as Admiral Nurses, we would always signpost those struggling with their grief to places they can seek further help.

Impact of COVID-19

As we have seen, when a person with dementia is told that someone close to them has died, it can be distressing. Some people will understand and experience grief, whereas others may not fully understand what this means, and this is often affected by their stage of dementia. People with dementia may have experienced several deaths during the COVID-19 pandemic (Duffy and Ballentine 2020) and the way to respond is no different to what we have described above.

Similarly, throughout the pandemic we have all had to adapt to guidance and restrictions that may have impacted upon visiting and how much time we have been able to spend with relatives who have contracted and subsequently died from COVID-19, both in hospitals and care homes. Although it is important to share the news as soon as possible, it also preferable to tell the person with dementia face to face. However, due to visiting restrictions, this may not always be possible due to only being able to make contact by telephone or virtually, using a video platform. If you do need to break such bad news by telephone or video call, it is advisable that, wherever possible, someone is with the person with dementia to help them to understand and offer support. The death of someone close is always hard. Helping someone with dementia to understand what has happened can be a daunting task, especially if you are grieving as well. Remember, you are only human, and you can only try your best. Hopefully, the advice and support offered in this chapter will help.

REFERENCES

Duffy, F. and Ballentine, J. (2020) 'Supporting a person with dementia following bereavement during the COVID-19 pandemic.' Northern Health and Social Care Trust. Accessed on 6/5/2020 at www.northerntrust.hscni.net/site/wp-content/uploads/2020/04/Supporting-a-person-with-Dementia-following-a-bereavement.pdf.

Feil, N. and De Klerk-Rubin, V. (2012) The Validation Breakthrough: Simple Techniques for Communicating with People with Alzheimer's and Other Dementias. Towson, MD: Health Professions Press.

Okada, A. and Matsuo, J. (2012) 'Emotional memory in patients with Alzheimer's disease: A report of two cases.' Case Reports in Psychiatry 2012, 313906. doi:10.1155/2012/313906.

Mace, N. and Rabins, P.V. (2021) The 36-Hour Day (7th edition). Baltimore, MD: Johns Hopkins University Press.

Mental Health Foundation (MHF) (2016) What is Truth? An Inquiry about Truth and Lying in Dementia Care. Accessed on 6/5/2020 at www.mentalhealth.org.uk/publications/what-truth-inquiry-about-truth-and-lying-dementia-care.

Watanbe, A. and Suwa, S. (2017) 'The mourning process of older people with dementia who lost their spouse.' Journal of Advanced Nursing 73, 9, 2143–2155. doi:10.1111/jan.13286.

RESOURCES AND FURTHER READING
Validation therapy

De Klerk-Rubin, V. (2008) *Validation Techniques for Dementia Care: The Family Guide to Improving Communication.* Towson, MD: Health Professions Press.

Validation therapy focuses on helping the person work through the emotions as a way to communicate, especially in people with dementia. See also:

https://best-alzheimers-products.com/validation-therapy-and-alzheimers.html

CRUSE Bereavement Support

CRUSE help people through one of the most painful times in life – with bereavement support and information.

www.cruse.org.uk

CHAPTER 13

'Time to go home now'

A STORY OF SUNDOWNING

Liz Murphy (pseudonym)

Mum, Sheila, is now 82 years old and got a diagnosis of vascular dementia three years ago. When Dad died, she came to live with me. Over the years, we have got on really well and settled into a lovely routine together, going to church, doing the gardening. It is only a small patch, but it suits us. Now things have changed, and as I am their only daughter and have no children of my own to fall back on, I am really struggling to cope. She spends most of the time walking about the house without a seemingly obvious purpose. The doctors have told me that she will need increasing amounts of care as it progresses. I really do not want her to go into a care home, but I am getting to the end of my tether. Mum seems to be in some sort of behaviour loop, and I have no idea how to deal with it.

From the minute she wakes, she is up and about; it is all I can do to contain her. She walks about continuously, following me around the house. I try to engage her in conversation, but she is very repetitive and generally replies with 'I am going to make a cup of tea'. Neverthe-less, when I make her a cup of tea, she doesn't really want it. I have tried distracting her, taking her back to her chair and giving her a magazine, but these things only settle her for a few minutes before she is up again. At some point in the afternoon, she does become more settled and will often fall asleep for a short while – I think she is exhausted. Then around teatime, she is up and off again. It's strange, but I can almost set my clock by the timing of her restlessness. The walking starts again after her nap, but she seems more agitated, and it becomes more as if she is pacing and getting faster. At this stage, Mum tries to get through any door, even opening cupboard doors, and seems to think this must be a way out. She says it's time for her to go now, but when I try to explain that she is home, she gets even more agitated and can even seem a bit aggressive when all I want to do is help. If I try to encourage her to sit down and join me doing something like watching the news, she resists me and can get even more agitated and angry with me. I cannot understand why she asks to go home as she has lived with me for the past 12 years, way before she had any signs of dementia. I love her so much, but I am becoming so tired. I have tried talking to the doctor, but he just says that it is 'part of her dementia', and he feels it is best if I now look at getting her into a care home as it's not going to get any better. He said that he does not want to give her any sedatives as they may make her wobbly and liable to fall.

SPECIALIST COMMENTARY

Dr Graham Stokes, Director of Memory Care Services, HC-One

What is the explanation for sundowning?
Sheila's need to walk throughout the day is not 'part of her dementia'. To see it in this way means falling prey to diagnostic overshadowing. In other words, much if not all that happens after the diagnosis of dementia is attributed to the diagnosis. There is no appreciation that a person's behaviour could be them expressing who they are; no consideration that the person might be reacting to their relationships and surroundings.

In part, the 'disease model' of dementia holds sway because its simplicity is seductive, but it is an explanation that provides neither solace nor solution. Instead, seeing Sheila's need to walk as 'part of who she is' does offer the possibility, if not probability, of mitigating or resolving Sheila's need to walk about the house.

During the day, I believe Sheila's repetitive reply 'I am going to make a cup of tea' does not truly reflect her wish for a cup of tea, for, as Liz says, when one is made for her, she doesn't really want it.

When asked by her daughter what she wants, Sheila has to say something and so she taps into her historical memories to come up with an everyday reason why she is walking around the house and says that she's going to make a cup of tea, for that's what she would have done innumerable times during her life. The clue as to what is motivating Sheila to walk continuously is Liz commenting that her mother is 'following me around the house'.

More going on here than sundowning

There are many needs that are met by walking 'to excess', each reflected in what the person with dementia is precisely doing. Sheila isn't simply walking continuously; she is staying close to Liz. Separation anxiety is the motivation and the need to be met. When Sheila is in the company of Liz, she is reassured and has peace of mind. Unfortunately, as Liz gets on with her life, Sheila cannot recall where her daughter has gone, how long she has been on her own, and, critically, she cannot remember anything that was said to reassure her that all is well, such as 'I'll be back in a minute'. Her daughter is just absent. Separation anxiety motivates Sheila to cling to Liz. The behaviour is known as 'trailing and tracking'. With this knowledge, we can suggest ways of being with Sheila that hold out the possibility that Liz may be able to help meet her mother's need to feel safe.

When Liz is busy around the house, she can make a bit of noise so she can be heard; leave doors open so her mother has good visual access; give Sheila brief boldly written notes explaining what she's doing and where she's gone. It may be possible to draw on simulated presence therapy (Abraha *et al.* 2020) which aims to simulate the presence of Liz by leaving Sheila with a family video or photo album (see also Chapter 1 on life story) that won't simply distract her but might absorb her. There are no guarantees of success, but having moved on from the 'disease model' of dementia, there are chances to mitigate Sheila's need to follow her daughter wherever she goes, and maybe Liz can gain a degree of comfort, and maybe even tolerance, knowing what is motivating her mother to walk continuously.

Sundowning

However, what is happening at teatime is different. Sheila is walking just as continuously but her manner is not the same. She is agitated, searching, wanting to go home, and gets angry. Sheila's behaviour is typical of sundowning, which presents as agitated, invasive walking that occurs at the end of the day and is characterised by a determination to search or leave. Again, as only a minority of people with dementia engage in this behaviour, we know we cannot simply accept the explanation that they do so 'because they have dementia'. Instead, we need to ask the question 'Why might someone with dementia become active and agitated as their day ends?'

We know that the brain damage in dementia can disrupt a person's sleep–wake cycle, but this would not explain Sheila's need to search or her agitation and saying 'it's time for her to go now' and asking to go home. From our earliest years, we are accustomed to 'leaving' as the day ends. We went home from nursery and school, college and work. Going somewhere at the end of the day is engrained within us, as is welcoming children and partners as they arrive home. For Sheila, as her day comes to an end, life begins to feel wrong. She says that 'it's time for her to go now', and the trigger for thinking this way is the changing atmosphere as dusk descends and evening preparations commence, such as preparing tea – as the sun downs.

Looking for meaning

This time, not only do we need to forensically reflect on Sheila's actions, but we also need to listen to the *meaning* that may lie behind her words. When Sheila asks to go home, she isn't referring to a place, a house or an address. It is not about bricks and mortar. If there is anyone who says what they don't mean, and means what they don't say, it is a person with dementia. Home is a metaphor that resonates with emotion. It is about being with family, to love and be loved; it is where you belong, to care and be cared for. It is that spot in your heart that says 'I'm safe'. It is these feelings that are motivating Sheila to ask to go home. Sheila's actions and words roll into one emotionally overwhelming need to know all is well, and as peace of mind eludes her, she becomes more and more agitated and angry.

As the past cannot be resurrected, and, as Liz says, she and her mother have lived together for 12 years, how might Liz calm and soothe her mother's troubled mind? Familiarity can help someone feel at peace. At the end of the day, her daughter might bring Sheila family photos to look at, or a treasured possession to touch and maybe talk about.

She might share memories about family and friends, always conversing in the past tense. Throughout, the golden thread for Liz is to be patient, listening to her mother's fears and frustrations as they keep resurfacing, and resisting the temptation to confront her with *our* reality ('when I try to explain that she is home') in a vain attempt to reassure her all is well, when Sheila knows it isn't. Liz also shouldn't be afraid to ask, 'What's the matter?' – the more she asks, the more she hears, which means the more she may understand what is upsetting her mother and how she may help her. A practical tip is, in the late afternoon and early evening, Liz could consider playing soothing music or relaxing sounds of nature to create a peaceful environment. Closing curtains and turning on lights before dusk can help. As can brightening the lights so the twilight and dusk of the end of the day is not so obvious.

Once more, we can see that an enriched understanding of dementia brings greater understanding and increases the likelihood that 'behaviours of concern' can be responded to in ways that have the potential to improve the lives of all affected by dementia. The underlying brain disease is not dismissed but the root-cause analysis when considering behaviours embraces the pathology of dementia, the person, their relationships and their life setting. Within this richness lies understanding and the prospect of change. Hope replaces despair, and positive approaches surface.

ADMIRAL NURSE ADVICE

Loraine Butterworth, Admiral Nurse, and
Dr Hilda Hayo, Chief Admiral Nurse

It is essential that we support Liz to understand where these problems may be coming from in relation to her mother's life history, physical health and stage of dementia – as Dr Stokes says, 'the root cause'. Importantly, it is also worth ruling out any underlying health issue that may be increasing Sheila's agitation, such as pain, dehydration, constipation, feeling unwell, change of medication – all of these may have an impact upon how she is feeling. Sometimes a person's wish to 'go home' is increased when they feel a need to 'get away' from something that is distressing them.

Simulation of presence

As Dr Stokes says, often the need to stay close to someone, in this case her daughter, has its origins in feeling insecure and needing to feel safe. Sheila feels that if she can keep Liz in eyesight, then all will be well; if Liz is there, then it lessens her sense of insecurity. The difficulty for Liz is that this might make her feel claustrophobic and that she is losing personal space. What can often help ease this pressure is to suggest that when, for example, a carer is performing a household task, they encourage the person with dementia to help, such as folding washing, sweeping the floor, dusting. In this case, helping may serve not only to reassure Sheila that her daughter is near and visible but also to provide a distraction while giving Sheila the opportunity to help, which could reduce anxiety and increase self-esteem. Of course, there will be times when Liz needs to go into another room or elsewhere. As Dr Stokes suggests, simulated presence therapy can help in reducing separation anxiety. Things to consider may be:

- Make a 'book of Liz' containing photographs of both Liz and her mother, so that Sheila can look through it and be reassured that Liz is well and healthy. This book can also be used to reminisce about their good life together and the lovely things that they have done.

- Liz could make some short films or voice recordings for her mother. These could include Liz talking as if to Sheila, reading something aloud to her mother (perhaps part of a favourite book or poem), videos of Liz doing everyday tasks around the house or out in the garden. Such things can simulate normal everyday life. These can be played when a carer is busy in another area of the house.

- Make a collage of yourself and the person with dementia using pictures in various rooms around the house (to reinforce a sense of familiarity by tying in people and places). A collage prepared on a piece of card to ensure durability is something that can be reached for easily.

- Another useful activity can be a collection of items of personal interest to the person with dementia, such as 'rummage' or memory boxes. So Sheila is presented with lots of reassuring images and items for her to see and feel. Such boxes can offer a distraction to a person's feelings of anxiety at being separated from their carer.

- Technology can also offer types of simulated presence, such as a talk back monitor – so in this case, Liz can continue chat to her mother even when they in different rooms, simulating her presence. Liz could be preparing a meal and talking to her mother at the same time. Sheila may find it comforting and reassuring to feel that Liz is 'present', and this might reduce her need to go and find her.

Past to present

There are various aspects of a person's past interests that can be used to enable them to feel emotionally secure in their environment. In Sheila's case, she had strong memories of her church life and a love of gardening. These can be used as ways to 'root' her to the home when she is walking around the house. This could be achieved by placing her favourite flowers and plants strategically around the house. Aromatic plants, such as herbs, add a further sensory experience because of their scent. Liz could make a gardening memory box for her mother that they could look through together while talking about plans for the garden, bulb planting, the flowers and plants Sheila loves.

When weather and seasons permit, Liz can spend time with Sheila in the garden, chatting about the flowers and plants there, and enable the connection with the flowers and plants strategically placed indoors. Time spent outside in the fresh air and daylight can feel calming and soothing for us all. This will offer an immediate form of engagement with Sheila, one that is less reliant upon her recall. This may also help with a natural flow for conversation, something Sheila finds a struggle.

A playlist of music that includes songs that have particular meaning for the person with dementia can also help when feeling insecure and the need to 'go home' arise. In Sheila's case, a music playlist may include her favourite hymns or organ recitals. Having hymn and prayer books, religious texts and pictures available in the house may help when Sheila is feeling uncertain, as would singing familiar hymns together, which may also provide some comfort.

Techniques that can help reduce distress

Some of the more distressing problems seem to occur after Sheila has woken from an afternoon nap. It may help if Liz tries to be there when her mother wakes up. This will have several potential benefits: time to have a cup of tea together, perhaps listening to her mother's music playlist or to looking through her memory box or life story book; a relaxing hand massage with scented oils may also help to relax Sheila. These are all ways that may help Sheila to reorientate herself following the nap and to feel safe and secure at this time of day. These activities may also help to reduce some of the distress and worry that people with dementia experience as the day wears on.

When a person with dementia becomes distressed, it is important to validate and acknowledge their feelings and not to immediately move to distraction. This may make them feel that you are not listening or taking their feelings seriously. Liz could validate her mother's feelings through actions and/or words to show an understanding and empathy for her mother's distress in wanting to 'go home'. For Sheila, to feel that Liz is on her side is important, which is less likely if Liz keeps telling her that she *is* home. Rather, Liz might talk to Sheila about her family home, describing what it was like and reminiscing about the times when she lived with her parents. This will move the conversation from unsafe ground, where her mother is trying to leave to 'go home', to safe ground, where her mother is talking of home and remembering home and the part it played in both their lives. Sometimes the person with dementia draws upon longer-term memories with more recent memories not accessible to them at that time. So if Liz can join her mother in sharing and talking about these longer-term memories, this may help.

Thinking about and planning for the future are important for families affected by dementia (see Chapter 5). As we see, in this case the GP suggests it is now time for full-time care, as 'it's not going to get any better'. We know that dementia is a progressive condition and will not 'get better', but our skills caring for and supporting a person with dementia can certainly 'get better', in that we can feel more equipped and able to provide support as time goes on. Caring for somebody with dementia can often feel as if you are standing on shifting sands, as the care needs of the person with dementia can seem to be continually changing; however, if we can better understand and adapt to these changes, this can make a huge difference. It is each family's own decision as to when, or if, full-time care is needed, as every family's circumstances are different. If a person does need to move into full-time care, then family carers can continue to support the person with dementia both during the transition and later in contributing to the planning and delivery of care (see Chapter 15). Family carers are the people who know the person with dementia best, often having a lifetime together.

REFERENCES

Abraha, I., Rimland, J.M., Lozano-Montoya, I., Dell'Aquila, G. *et al.* (2020) 'Simulated presence therapy for dementia (review).' *Cochrane Database of Systematic Reviews 2020*, 4, CD011882. doi:10.1002/14651858.CD011882.pub3.

RESOURCES AND FURTHER READING

Khachiyants, N., Trinkle, D., Joon Son, S. and Kim, K.Y. (2011) 'Sundown syndrome in persons with dementia: An update.' *Psychiatry Investigation 8*, 4, 275–287. doi:10.4306/pi.2011.8.4.275.

Peak, J.S. and Cheston, R. (2002) 'Using simulated presence therapy with people with dementia.' *Ageing and Mental Health 6*, 1, 77–81. doi:10.1080/13607860120101095.

Stokes, G. (1996) 'Challenging Behaviour in Dementia: A Psychological Approach.' In R. Woods (ed.) *Clinical Psychology of Ageing*. Chichester: John Wiley.

Stokes, G. (2000) *Challenging Behaviour in Dementia: A Person-Centred Approach.* Bicester: Winslow Press.

Stokes, G. (2008) *And Still the Music Plays: Stories of People with Dementia*. London: Hawker Publications.

Dementia UK

SUNDOWNING

www.dementiauk.org/get-support/understanding-changes-in-dementia/sundowning

COPING WITH DISTRESS

www.dementiauk.org/wp-content/uploads/2022/03/V5_DUKFS22_Coping-with-distress-NEW.pdf

Pictures to Share

Pictures to Share books provide an enjoyable way of maintaining meaningful communication with someone who may be hard to reach.

www.picturestoshare.co.uk

Assistive technology in dementia: talk back monitors

Assistive technology devices and systems that help people maintain or improve their independence, safety, and wellbeing at home.

www.scie.org.uk/dementia/support/housing/assistive-technology

CHAPTER 14

'Why is it so complicated?'

NHS CONTINUING HEALTHCARE FUNDING

Brian Humphreys

Our problems were centred around Jane's unpredictable aggression. While I had got used to being the focus of her aggression, it became a different matter when Jane started being violent to her carers. In September 2020, I introduced carers to Jane for just an hour every morning to see how it went. After a few weeks, once everything appeared to have settled down, I wanted to go out with the local running club on their training night, and so organised for the carers to come for two hours on Thursday nights and give me my first taste of 'freedom' in a long while. While out running, I got a phone call and had to return home to a very distressed carer on the doorstep who had been scratched, her hair pulled, choked and her earring pulled out. It was a very traumatic experience for her. Seeing her like this made me realise what I had been going through and had just brushed off. The care agency was fantastic and tried numerous ways to help me, but in the end, they had to refuse to send anyone out unless I was also going to be in the house. I was desperate for help to allow me to have some kind of life outside the confines of the home.

It was suggested to me by our Admiral Nurse that Jane might be eligible for NHS continuing healthcare (CHC) funding, and that it would be worth applying. I first contacted the memory clinic and asked our community mental health nurse (CMHN) if she would be able to start the process. She came around to the house to do the initial checklist which was a very painless process.

The second thing I did was to go online and download the

National Framework for CHC and the Decision Support Tool (DST), both of which are very important to read and understand. However, I found that the complexities of the DST take a long time to get your head around, particularly understanding the interactions between care domains and the need to understand and explain the intensity and complexity of the needs.

The CHC assessment was held via a telephone conference because we were in the middle of the COVID pandemic. The DST is supposed to be a multi-disciplinary team consisting of the CHC assessor, someone who understands the patient and a social worker. The first attempt at doing the DST consisted of a direct phone call to myself; when I asked if they had arranged for others to attend, I was told that they had not, so I asked for the meeting to be postponed until it could have the correct attendees.

I telephoned our social worker to ask if she would join the meeting and was told that she had just had a phone call with the CHC assessor afterwards. I phoned our CMHN and Admiral Nurse, and managed to secure the Admiral Nurse for the next call.

I felt as though the initial DST assessment was deliberately focused on keeping the attendees as few as possible (just two of us), which would give a completely unbalanced and potentially biased result because the DST process and scoring is relatively complex and only the CHC assessor on the call understands the process fully.

Having our Admiral Nurse on the call was an absolute godsend. She understood the process as well as the CHC assessor did, and knew which elements of Jane's condition should be aimed at which care domain and how to describe the complexities and intensities.

Despite the preparation I had made in advance of the meeting, I did have the strong feeling that the CHC assessor was being obstructive in the scoring of Jane's condition. Despite my inability to organise any kind of social care for Jane so that I could leave the house, and despite having various safeguarding reports and care agency incident reports, the CHC assessor would only rate Jane's challenging behaviour as 'high' and not 'severe'.

However, subsequent to the DST meeting and a change of assessor at the CHC, the initial scoring was overruled, and Jane's challenging behaviour was rated as severe without any intervention from me. That was a nice surprise and restored my faith in the system.

The best thing to come out of being awarded CHC is that decisions on how to provide care for Jane have been taken out of my hands. It was now the responsibility of the NHS to find an agency that would be willing and able to take on the complex care needs for Jane and develop a care prescription that considered not just Jane's needs but my own.

I have been able to develop a relationship with the Senior CHC Nurse Specialist to talk through our care needs, to change and enhance the care prescription, and add in additional hours. Additionally, due to Jane's rapid decline, she has also been extremely helpful in identifying potential care homes that we could research ready for when that time comes, so that we're making an informed decision rather than a rushed one.

SPECIALIST COMMENTARY

Jo-Ann Dawson, Admiral Nurse, Central
Norfolk Admiral Nurse Service

What is NHS continuing healthcare funding?

NHS continuing healthcare (CHC) funding is a package of ongoing care that is arranged and funded solely by the NHS. It is for adults with long-term, complex and unpredictable health needs which are above and beyond what can be met by social care. Social care needs include managing personal hygiene, toileting, nutrition and ensuring a person is appropriately dressed, whereas health needs are to ensure the treatment, control, management and prevention of disease, illness, injury or disability. However, these areas of care can overlap and cause confusion. Normally, NHS healthcare is free, but CHC covers other costs such as home carers or care home fees. CHC may be awarded if the person is assessed as having a 'primary health need' – that is, if dealing with health issues is the most important part of their care. However, there are exceptions to this in certain circumstances, such as when conditions involve changes to behaviours.

In essence, this means that CHC is available to people who meet certain eligibility criteria, across England, Wales and Northern Ireland, and who require significant, ongoing *healthcare* outside of the hospital environment. In Scotland, CHC has been replaced by a scheme called Hospital Based Complex Clinical Care; this funding is only available to people who need to be in hospital to have their healthcare needs met. However, in Scotland personal and nursing care is free for those who have been assessed as eligible, and a person can claim personal care and nursing care payments to cover those elements of care home fees.

Continuing healthcare assessment process
STAGE ONE - THE CHC CHECKLIST

The CHC assessment is a two-stage process. The first stage requires a CHC checklist to be completed. The checklist is a screening tool, which has an intentionally low threshold to ensure that all of those people who are potentially eligible for assessment are given the opportunity to participate in the process. The checklist should be completed by a health or social care professional who has been appropriately trained to complete the assessment.

The checklist assesses 11 domains for care (see box) and is designed to be quick and straightforward to complete.

NHS CHC CHECKLIST - 11 DOMAINS OF CARE

- Breathing
- Nutrition
- Continence
- Skin integrity
- Mobility
- Communication
- Psychological/emotional
- Cognition
- Behaviour
- Drug therapies and medication
- Altered states of consciousness

In each domain the assessor will decide if the person's needs are high (A), moderate (B) or low/no needs (C). A full assessment will be triggered if:

- two or more areas are rated A

- five or more areas are rated B, or one A and four Bs

- there is an A rating in any of: behaviour, breathing, drug therapies and medication, or altered states of consciousness.

Once the checklist has been completed, there are two possible outcomes:

- The person *is* put forward for a full assessment of need.

- The person *is not* put forward for a full assessment of need.

If the threshold is met for a full assessment of need, the person should be assessed using the Decision Support Tool (DST) within 28 days.

STAGE TWO – FULL ASSESSMENT OF NEED: DECISION SUPPORT TOOL (DST)

In order to complete a full assessment of need, the CHC assessor should complete a DST. The information to complete the DST can be gathered from medical and care notes, professional observations, and also the observations of those providing care for the person being assessed. The person and/or their representatives are in a good position to provide up-to-date and timely evidence for the assessment. The CHC assessor may hold the meeting and assessment face to face or by video/tele conferencing, but whichever method is selected, they should ensure active participation of all members as far as possible. The full assessment of need and DST meeting should be arranged by the CHC assessor so that there is full involvement of the person being assessed, where mental capacity allows, and/or their representative. Also present should be any members of the health and social care team who are actively involved with the person being assessed to ensure that information and evidence of the person's care needs are accurately presented in the DST. The CHC assessor has the responsibility for coordinating and completing the full assessment of need and the DST.

The DST consists of the domains indicated in the box above and an additional one requesting that 'other significant care needs to be taken into consideration'. The DST assessment offers a framework to enable the gathering of evidence to highlight the overall level of health need. This is achieved by considering the domains of care and also by establishing the nature, complexity, intensity and unpredictability level of the health need.

The CHC assessor should seek the person and/or their representative's agreement of the content of the assessment and the level of need identified across the domains. If concerns or disagreements arise, the CHC assessor should try to address these at the assessment and document any disagreements.

WHAT HAPPENS ONCE THE DST IS COMPLETED?

Once the DST has been completed, a recommendation is made to the local NHS body responsible for awarding funding as to whether the person is eligible for CHC. Only in very rare circumstances can the local NHS body overrule this recommendation. A letter will be sent to explain whether or not CHC funding has been awarded. If CHC has been awarded, a CHC nurse should work with the person (or designated carer) to devise a support plan which will include:

- the person's health and wellbeing goals

- the day-to-day care and support they need

- how their needs and care will be managed

- where their care will be provided (e.g. in their own home or a care home)

- who will be responsible for providing their care.

CHC funding can either be paid directly to the person's care service provider or as a Personal Health Budget. The Personal Health Budget is usually managed by a family member, health and social care professional or care organisation, and gives more control and flexibility over how the funding is used.

WHAT HAPPENS IF THE PERSON DOES NOT QUALIFY FOR CHC?

If a person and/or their representative do not agree with the outcome of a DST assessment and/or a subsequent review, there is an appeal process. Details of how to appeal should be given at the close of the

DST assessment; this is usually done by informing the individual that a formal outcome letter will be sent following a review of the assessment recommendations by a panel which will also include how to appeal the process/outcome.

If the person's CHC application is found to be ineligible for full NHS CHC funding, but elements of their care indicate a health need, they may be eligible for NHS funded nursing care (FNC) if they are residing in a care home with nursing.

It is important to remember that a person's needs can change, and the assessment may need to be reconsidered. This would be done by revisiting the previous assessment and carrying out a further DST assessment.

NHS CHC fast-track funding

If a person's health needs are rapidly deteriorating and it is considered they are approaching the end of their life, then eligibility for NHS fast-track funding could be considered if they have a primary health need. This funding is aimed at ensuring people have quick access to NHS CHC funding, without the need to participate in the DST assessment process. Completing the NHS fast-track tool requires an appropriate clinician, such as a GP, consultant, registrar or registered nurse who has experience and knowledge of the person's needs, to evidence that a person has a rapidly deteriorating condition and may be entering the terminal stage of their condition. It is important that eligibility is not determined by expected length of life remaining but by need.

This section has served to offer an overview, raise awareness and enable a basic understanding of the NHS CHC process and the key elements that should be adhered to. However, given the complex nature of the process and how it relates to people with dementia, it is important that families are fully informed and, where possible, get the right advice and information. There are lots of organisations that can advocate and offer independent advice, guidance and support to help people with dementia and their families to navigate this complicated assessment and funding system (see the 'Resources and further reading' section at the end of this chapter).

ADMIRAL NURSE ADVICE

Zena Aldridge, Admiral Nurse
Research Fellow, Dementia UK

Lack of awareness of CHC and its purpose

Organising care for a person with dementia can be a difficult process, which affects families at times when they are feeling stressed and vulnerable. Sadly, Jane's story is an all too familiar one. I have worked with many families who were unaware of the existence of NHS CHC or who have struggled to successfully navigate the process. The lack of awareness of what CHC is, what it is for and how to get an assessment is a significant problem, with a further challenge being the lack of clarity when trying to distinguish between health and social care needs. It is not only people with dementia and their families who lack awareness; in my experience, very few health and social care professionals have a clear understanding of dementia and its effects, the CHC process and when it is relevant to people living with dementia.

Cracks in the pathway

There are a multitude of issues that impact negatively on the ability of families to succeed in obtaining CHC. However, the lack of awareness about CHC and how it relates to people with dementia is not surprising, given that services for people affected by dementia are often fragmented, which, sadly, allows people to slip through gaps in the system. Health and social care professionals may not always consider the person with dementia and their family's needs in totality or holistically. Often, the person is viewed from the perspective of a singular, disease-oriented approach which may be a reflection of a lack of understanding of the impact of dementia. It must not always be assumed that people working in dementia services (e.g. community mental health teams) are fully versed in the wider needs of people with dementia.

While, historically, dementia care has been firmly sited within mental health services, a report by the Nuffield Council on Bioethics (2009) redefined dementia as a brain disease, not a mental health problem. Yet it is still the case that dementia is perceived differently from other brain diseases. This is evident in Jane's case. Despite Jane being under the care of a community mental health nurse (CMHN) and displaying distressed behaviours, which could be considered a priority domain in the CHC checklist, the CMHN had not suggested that Jane might be eligible for CHC. It may be that the CMHN had been focusing on trying to identify the cause of the behaviour and manage it from a mental health perspective, rather than considering the wider impact of the behaviour on Jane, her husband and those who cared for her.

Lack of quality and consistency of the CHC process
When considering the National Framework for NHS continuing healthcare and NHS-funded nursing care (Department of Health and Social Care 2018) in relation to this case study, it is clear that the appropriate processes and procedures had been disregarded, starting right at the beginning with the lack of information about the process. It is the role of the CHC assessor/coordinator to ensure the process is explained fully, that information is provided and the National NHS CHC framework is followed. Despite clear processes and guidance for professionals, there is still a lack of consistency in the manner in which they are interpreted. The NHS CHC framework clearly states that the person and/or their representatives should be informed and provided with information regarding the process, and that their participation and consent should be actively sought, which does not appear to be the case for Jane's family.

The DST assessment should be based on the evidence and assessment of need, with all those present at the assessment being able to contribute to providing that evidence. The focus should be to highlight the level of need across the DST domains to ensure the correct support and funding is provided in a timely manner.

This would be difficult to achieve in Jane's DST assessment as it was attempted without the presence of a full multi-disciplinary team (MDT). Individual phone calls do not constitute an MDT discussion, nor do they enable an opportunity to share evidence and have transparent discussions about a person's level of need. While the COVID-19 pandemic and lockdown/isolation measures have created obstacles in conducting face-to-face MDT discussions, the CHC framework is very clear in stating that the DST assessment can be undertaken face to face by using video/teleconferencing. Sadly, there does not appear to have been an attempt to offer this in Jane's case.

The importance of specialist dementia support and expertise

In Jane's case, it was an Admiral Nurse who first suggested that a CHC checklist should be completed by looking at the situation and encouraging the family to ask for this to be done, and it was the Admiral Nurse who ensured they were better informed about the CHC process. The Admiral Nurse was able to use their specialist clinical knowledge to ensure the correct information was provided at the revisited DST assessment and enable appropriate articulation of Jane's needs and how they related to the assessment domains. All of this positively impacted on the outcome of the assessment. Yet not all families are able to access this type of specialist support and so it is imperative that families are aware of organisations that can offer specialist support and guidance. The presence of someone with specialist knowledge regarding dementia at the DST MDT can support not only the family of the person being assessed but also other members of the MDT who may have limited knowledge of dementia and its effects.

It important to recognise that the CHC process can be applied to people with a multitude of conditions, and it cannot be assumed that the CHC nurse assessor will be an expert in dementia care. The needs of people with dementia can often be complex, and there is a known lack of skills and knowledge about dementia and its effects across health and social care systems.

Aside from the issues highlighted in the case study, the CHC process is fraught with challenges for people with dementia, their families and carers. The manner in which a primary health need is defined can make it difficult for people with dementia to be approved for CHC. The DST assessment domains are the same for all conditions, and they do not therefore intuitively represent the needs of all conditions equitably.

Consequently, the assessment and its outcome are very much dependent on the professional conducting the assessment, their interpretation of needs and attributing evidence to the correct domains to weight scoring appropriately. Thus, it is essential to involve specialist dementia expertise in the MDT to improve outcomes for families affected by dementia.

In summary

Getting the right care for a person with dementia, whether it be health or social care, can be fraught with challenges, and therefore it is important that families access specialist advice and support where possible. Although not all families will have access to local Admiral Nurse Services, there are organisations that can offer support and guidance (see the 'Resources and further reading' section at the end of this chapter).

To help you through the process, Jo-Ann and I have a few top tips to help you:

- Always seek support, information and/or guidance from an organisation that knows about dementia and the CHC process.

- Don't assume that all health and social care professionals understand dementia or the CHC process. If you think the person you are caring for is eligible, ask for a checklist to be considered.

- If you are unsure about anything, ask questions. If you don't agree, you are able to offer a challenge.

- Make sure you have the contact details of the CHC coordinator, that you receive a copy of the checklist and a blank copy of the DST assessment document before the MDT so you can write notes and prepare.

- Evidence is key, so keeping a note of some of your concerns or recording events that you feel are important in demonstrating the needs of the person with dementia is important. You can give a copy of your notes to the CHC coordinator.

- Make sure you have information about the appeals process and organisations that can help you with advocacy services if you later need support in making an appeal.

- If the person with dementia isn't eligible for continuing healthcare, seek guidance on what other support they may be entitled to meet their needs.

REFERENCES

Department of Health and Social Care (2018) 'NHS continuing healthcare checklist.' Accessed on 9/5/2022 at https://assets.publishing.service.gov.uk/government/uploads/system/uploads/attachment_data/file/783048/continuing_healthcare_checklist_-_December_2018_revised.odt.

Department of Health and Social Care (2018) 'NHS continuing healthcare decision support tool.' Accessed on 9/5/2022 at www.gov.uk/government/publications/nhs-continuing-healthcare-decision-support-tool.

Department of Health and Social Care (2018) 'NHS continuing healthcare fast-track pathway tool.' Accessed on 9/5/2022 at www.gov.uk/government/publications/nhs-continuing-healthcare-fast-track-pathway-tool.

Department of Health and Social Care (2018) 'NHS continuing healthcare public information leaflet.' Accessed on 9/5/2022 at https://assets.publishing.service.gov.uk/government/uploads/system/uploads/attachment_data/file/770684/National_framework_for_CHC_and_FNC_-_public_information_leaflet.pdf.

Department of Health and Social Care (2018) 'National Framework for NHS continuing healthcare and NHS-funded nursing care.' Accessed on 9/5/2022 at https://assets.publishing.service.gov.uk/government/uploads/system/uploads/attachment_data/file/746063/20181001_National_Framework_for_CHC_and_FNC_-_October_2018_Revised.pdf.

Nuffield Council on Bioethics (2009) 'Dementia: Ethical issues.' Accessed on 9/5/2022 at www.nuffieldbioethics.org/publications/dementia.

RESOURCES AND FURTHER READING

Reddall, C. (2021) *Anna and the Beast: The True Story of a Young Mum Diagnosed with Dementia, Aged 37*. Cheltenham: Goldcrest Books International. Chapter 14, especially pp.100–101 (where CHC funding is discussed).

Age UK

Age UK (2021) 'NHS continuing healthcare and NHS-funded nursing care factsheet FS20.' Available at: www.ageuk.org.uk/globalassets/age-uk/documents/factsheets/fs20_nhs_continuing_healthcare_and_nhs-funded_nursing_care_fcs.pdf.

Age UK Advice (England) 0800 169 65 65

Age Cymru Advice (Wales) 0300 303 4498

Age NI (Northern Ireland) 0808 8080 7575

Age Scotland (Scotland) 0800 124 4222

Alzheimer's Society

Alzheimer's Society (2019) 'When does the NHS pay for care? How to apply for NHS continuing healthcare funding in England and how to appeal if it is not awarded.' Accessed on 9/5/2022 at www.alzheimers.org.uk/sites/default/files/migrate/downloads/when_does_the_nhs_pay_for_care.pdf.

Dementia UK

Dementia UK (2021) 'Guide to continuing healthcare (CHC) funding.' Accessed on 9/5/2022 at www.dementiauk.org/get-support/legal-and-financial-information/guide-to-continuing-healthcare-funding.

CHAPTER 15

'I just felt as though I had failed her when she needed me most'

TRANSITION INTO A CARE HOME

Alan Hewitt

I am a former carer for my wife who was diagnosed with dementia. She lived for five years after she was diagnosed. I could cope with everything that dementia threw at me as long as I knew what was happening. It was when things happened that I had no control over that made it so hard. A few months before Ann died, I was diagnosed with bowel cancer and was admitted to hospital for surgery. Being diagnosed with bowel cancer didn't bother me in the slightest. What bothered me was that Ann would have to spend eight weeks in a nursing home as I was advised that this would be the shortest time that it would take me to recover from the surgery.

As it turned out, I wasn't well enough to have Ann home after the eight weeks. While hanging out washing for the first time, I collapsed in the garden. I had to extend Ann's stay in the nursing home in order for me to recuperate further. I felt so guilty knowing that I wasn't strong enough to look after her. Ann started to deteriorate, and during the last four weeks of her life, she was hardly eating or drinking. She seemed to have shut down. Her chin was down on her chest the whole of the time and I couldn't get her to react to anything. I wondered if she thought I had abandoned her. I felt so guilty and depressed. I used sit in my car after leaving her and cry. I would have given anything to get her home. If I had known that this was going to happen, I wouldn't have had the cancer operation. I just felt as though I had failed her when she needed me most.

The guilt will live with me forever

Sylvia Bates

Mum was diagnosed at the age of 68. We were just told her brain scan showed signs of her brain dying and that she had dementia, and then we were left to get on with life. Mum did not appear to understand, and as she was fiercely independent, it was very difficult to help her. She slowly admitted to difficulties with managing her bills, so I took over the banking and shopping. Sadly, I didn't always understand how to react to the changes that were happening to Mum and feel now that I didn't always do and say the right things. One such memory stays with me. It was the day after my son's wedding. Mum came round all excited having just walked into town and bought a pair of white diamanté pumps. She thought they would be perfect for the wedding. I said, 'The wedding was yesterday, Mum.' Her face fell as she realised what I had said. I will never forget that look, and wish I had just replied that the shoes were lovely.

When Mum's elder sister was admitted into care with dementia, Mum said to me, 'I never want to go into a care home. I would rather you help me kill myself than be trapped inside dementia. If ever I lack capacity, please do the kindest act for me and free me.' She kept a large stock of medication at home and always said that she would take an overdose if she thought she would ever become a burden on anyone.

Over the next seven years, I experienced many problems. I became embarrassed by Mum's appearance, having gone from a smart, beautiful woman to a 'bag lady'. Smelly, hair not brushed and wearing the same clothes for days on end until I could wrestle her into the bath and get her clothes into the washing machine. One Saturday, we had heated words over this, whereupon mum walked out of the house. After about half an hour, she returned and hugged me. We both cried and she said she couldn't manage without me. I promised her I would always be there for her and that it wasn't a problem, as I loved her. That is the last memory I have of a 'real' conversation with my mum.

Mum went to stay with one of my siblings so I could take a much-needed holiday. I felt so guilty leaving her, but I needed the break. Things did not go well and I was bombarded with calls saying they were unable to cope with Mum. I finally contacted social services for help. They sent in carers, which Mum hated. She used to hide under the bed or she would get up and go out to avoid them. She was angry with me for arranging this care. In the last six months at home, things got worse. The realisation hit me when, on a snowy, cold February night around 11pm, she came to my door wearing just a silky nightie and wrap. That was the night I fell to pieces. I realised that I could not cope anymore and that Mum would have to go into care. I was going to do the very thing that she asked me not to. I rang emergency social care but they were not interested, so I had to wait until the Monday to phone social services and arrangements were made for Mum to go into the psychiatric unit for assessment. I could not be the one take her in and then leave her. I knew she would kick off, so an ambulance was arranged to take her. I sat at home crying, racked with guilt.

Mum didn't go quietly, and the police had to be called as she became violent and out of control and had to be sectioned. I now feel so guilty for putting my own fears before my mum. Maybe things would have been different if I had gone with her? As suspected, the outcome of her assessment was that she should be put into care. I cried and cried, knowing my mum would rather be dead than have this. I did what I had to do and found a care home. It looked lovely, and Mum settled in surprisingly well.

The guilt didn't stop there, though; I felt guilty that I couldn't visit her every day. On the days I did visit, Mum would often be soiled and wet and dressed in someone else's clothes. It was obvious to me that she was not getting the care she deserved. The final straw was when I found an unreported bedsore on Mum. Mum was moved into another care home, but this one was no better. After many complaints and meetings, I was again looking for another home. The guilt I felt at not being able to look after her at home was unbearable, compounded by the fact that I hadn't found a good care home. I felt so guilty for letting my mum down.

The final home was better, but by this time Mum could not walk, and she didn't really talk to family members from the day she went into this home. The staff used to say she would talk with them. Wow, did that hurt! It felt as though she was punishing me for putting her in a home. This only served to further fuel my guilt. I felt guilty when I didn't visit, but it broke my heart to see her every time I did visit. I prayed for seven years that Mum would die so that her suffering would stop. How could you wish that your mum was dead? I did. Mum died aged 81. Sorry, my darling mum, that you had to go through this. I put you in a home and I could do nothing to stop your suffering. You did not get the care you deserved and the guilt will live with me forever.

I had promised I would always look after her

Theresa Clarke

My mother lived with my husband and me for 24 years. She was a very active and clever person who enjoyed a varied social life and helped me out around the home, which was great as we both worked full-time. When mum turned 80, she started to say things out of character and use swear words, which was something she had never done. She was eventually diagnosed with vascular dementia and almost overnight her condition deteriorated. She began to see things that weren't there and turned quite violent towards me, which led to an admission to a psychiatric hospital for an assessment. I hated visiting her in that place, but worst of all was having to leave without her. She used to cling on to my arm, pleading with me to take her home, yet at the same time swearing and punching out at me.

Although deep down I knew she would never come back home, the guilt I felt at not being able to look after and take care of her went deep to my core. I had promised I would always look after her, and now I felt I had betrayed her and let her down. Although many professionals had told me it was for the best and I would never be able to handle her, that feeling of utter betrayal has never left me.

Mum was transferred to a nursing home, and over the next four years, I watched as she gradually deteriorated: the dramatic weight loss, the incontinence, the inability to hold a conversation and finally the inability to recognise me. I thought it was my punishment for not keeping my promise to her. I must have shed enough tears over the five years until she died to fill an ocean. I did, however, keep my promise in the end when I went and collected her ashes: I brought her home.

SPECIALIST COMMENTARY

Jill Manthorpe, Professor of Social Work, King's College London

It is sad to read these three accounts but important to recognise that they do not cover every family carers' experiences and there is probably a very great spectrum of feelings among family and friends who make the decision about moving their relative to a care home and then take on a different role in their lives. The commentary from the Admiral Nurse below sets out some of the ways in which living with guilt can be managed by reframing the decision and also some ways of not dwelling on the decision but making the most of this new chapter in everyone's lives.

For many people, the image of care homes compounds their feelings that they are not doing their best by even considering a move. Many people are frightened by the very idea, especially if they remember the workhouse and long-stay geriatric wards and think care homes are pretty similar. Others might say that, in their culture, it is almost shameful to have an older family member in a care home. While most older people do want to stay at home as long as possible, moving to a care home can be a positive choice, especially if it involves moving to a home where staff, activities and routines are already known. In our study of short respite stays in a care home, we found that they not only provided a valuable break but helped everyone concerned to see if the care home was welcoming and if it might provide a long-term option if things changed at home (Samsi, Cole and Manthorpe 2021).

Such decisions were not made lightly but often were the result of an accumulation of stressors, exhausting other care options, followed a risk/benefit analysis and took into consideration the wishes of person with dementia and their readiness to move. As the three personal accounts illustrate, for some the idea of a 'tipping point' being reached reflected their experiences. But some felt strongly that early planning, prior experiences of care homes or one particular care home, understanding funding arrangements and having support with decision making did help or would have helped. Interestingly, in our study, the care home manager or administrator often seemed to be the most helpful in terms of explaining costs and payments – especially if the person with dementia was not eligible for local authority funding (Samsi *et al.* 2021).

The pandemic effect on care homes

Of course, the COVID-19 pandemic has changed our ideas about whether care homes are safe places and whether a move to a care home might mean visiting is very restricted. It is hard to generalise about this, but there have been specific moves (at the time of writing) that enable relatives to be 'essential care givers' – not necessarily to provide care but to offer the family connections and companionship that can help residents stay well. This is a new public health perspective which acknowledges the risk of harm of isolation from visitors on the physical and mental health of residents, specifically distress, loneliness and accelerated cognitive decline.

Like many services during the pandemic, things changed in many care homes, such as greater use of online communications to keep in touch with relatives. This will be welcomed by many family carers. Although it means that some will need to get online and develop the skills to become familiar with this form of communication, going forward it can add a further resource for keeping in touch. And relatives of care home residents have become more powerful advocates for their rights, with groups such as the Relatives & Residents Association and Rights for Residents (see the 'Resources and further reading' section at the end of this chapter) emphasising that people in care homes and their relatives have human rights. Both these organisations can take up individual concerns and are a good source of information and support.

Nonetheless, we need to acknowledge that care homes were not well supported during the COVID-19 pandemic – an international problem of lack of attention, little involvement in disaster or pandemic planning and preparedness, and insufficient resources (see Collateral Global 2021).

While our focus as relatives or friends is likely to be on one individual, there are major problems that need to be resolved by policy makers. For care home staff, it has been very distressing to witness the deaths from COVID-19 and the associated 'excess deaths' (probably undiagnosed COVID-19 but also from other health problems) during this period (Wu *et al.* 2021). Both care home staff and residents need to be better supported in the future, and both will need the backing of residents' families to make this possible.

Changing perceptions of care homes

COVID-19 has also perhaps changed some of society's ideas about care homes and care home workers and what they provide. While the social care sector has been arguing for many years that the system of funding for care is woefully inadequate and that this sector of care is stigmatised, it seems to have taken the pandemic to make more people appreciate that care homes and care home workers provide essential support, and that while they may be low paid, they are certainly not low skilled. Indeed, care home workers can often offer suggestions about how to make the move less stressful and when might be the best time to make the move (Samsi *et al.* 2021).

What might be the alternatives to a care home?

The three accounts above illustrate how some family carers struggle alone and how, even if they try to bring in outside help – such as Sylvia who contacted her local authority for help – this does not always work. Homecare does work for many people, however, even up to the end of life. There are several sources of advice about getting an assessment from the local authority's social services or social care department, such as the Admiral Nurse Dementia Helpline or the Alzheimer's Society, and these often mention that there are now several ways of getting help in the home. For example, some homecare agencies specialise in dementia care, and their caregivers may be very familiar with the difficulties that Sylvia encountered. Other options include directly employing a homecare worker oneself – either paying from one's own or family's income and savings or getting money from the local authority to do this (a personal budget or direct payment). While this can mean taking on some administrative work, in several areas there are organisations that will take this on. Employing someone directly provides continuity and a bit more flexibility as they may do a range of tasks with the person with dementia and/or for them.

Research shows that these arrangements can suit families very well (Manthorpe *et al.* 2021). At times, the caregiver was able to provide support for wider members of the family, and when things worked well, these directly employed caregivers and family members were forming in effect a care team, characterised by mutual trust and close working. For some people, such options can help provide support that is culturally acceptable – for example, same-sex personal care or provision of food and drink that reflects a person's preferences or habits.

Similarly, while not for everyone, other options include employing a live-in caregiver which may be preferred to moving to a care home. There is a range of homecare agencies that offer this option as well as people who make their own private arrangements. Like everything, there are advantages and disadvantages of taking this route, but again for some families they work well (Vandrevala and O'Dwyer 2022). Such arrangements can be time-limited – for example, if a family carer needs a break but does not think their family member wants to move or would adjust well in a new setting – or they can be for as long as suits one or both parties. Discussion with the homecare agency about mutual expectations and financial arrangements will help clarify if this might be an option.

Such alternatives can work and a care home might never be needed. If it does become necessary, a care home move is not a failure, and as the Admiral Nurses below describe, it can be in the best interests of everyone or one person. Ideally, people will have talked about possible futures after a dementia diagnosis or as part of general discussions about getting older (see Chapter 5). But for some people, the time is never right or they get overtaken by events. Advance care planning can assist, but as the three accounts from carers above illustrate, they can lead to promises that are hard to keep, as Theresa mentions and as Sylvia alludes to in saying she will always be there for her mother. Professionals need to listen out for these memorable conversation reports when undertaking their assessments and reviews. Their skills lie in helping to understand what lies behind such promises and acknowledging the strengths of the relationship and how these can be sustained whatever the living arrangements. As with many social situations it may be that sharing this with others who are similarly affected can be doubly supportive – hence the common advice from professionals to join family carers' groups in person or online. Online groups can also have the advantage of offering opportunities for family carers in different circumstances to share their views and experiences, whether they are same-sex groups, family carers or people with different forms of dementia (early onset, for example) or from different cultural or ethnic backgrounds. Carers' organisations and new professionals working in dementia care such as social prescribers are likely to be good sources of such information, as well as specialist dementia professionals, such as Admiral Nurses.

ADMIRAL NURSE ADVICE

Rachael Lowe, Admiral Nurse, Dementia UK, and **Saul Mason**, Admiral Nurse Regional Lead, Royal British Legion

Feelings of guilt

Guilt is a common feeling experienced by many family carers when caring for someone with dementia. It may be feelings of guilt for being embarrassed about odd behaviours, for losing your temper, for wishing you did not have the responsibility of care or for moving the person you care for into a home.

Caring for someone with dementia can force us to make decisions, such as stopping them from driving, which, when in better health, the person would have been fully able to decide for themselves. All this can add to feelings of guilt. People also feel guilt for reasons they don't always understand. Being a family carer may be objectively achievable for a few days, weeks and perhaps even months, but family carers of people with dementia are often undertaking caring for years. That is plenty of time for guilt to grow and fester.

Going into a care home

As Professor Manthorpe describes, the term 'care home' can have negative connotations for many people, but a good care home might be the best option for a person with dementia. Sometimes, when family carers place the person with dementia in a good care home, they may observe that the person seems to thrive and appear better than they did at home. This may be because people with dementia often benefit from the routine of a care home or the additional company. However, even such a change for the better can bring up feelings of guilt that this could not be achieved at home. Alternatively, there may be a sense of relief that the burden of care has been lifted. All these feelings can be in conflict with each other, which adds to an increased sense of guilt.

Lost routines

When I worked in a nursing home, family carers often told me that they felt lost without the usual routine and demands of caring for the person with dementia at home. They didn't know what to do with themselves and couldn't seem to relax. For some, the trips to the care home were tiring, especially when the distance between home and the care home was great. Some family carers found it depressing to visit, seeing other residents in the care home with greater needs than their family members. When first moving to a care home, a person with dementia may seem to deteriorate, and family carers might perceive this is their fault for instigating the move. However, after a period of adjustment to the new setting, this downward turn can start to improve. Nevertheless, this period of change can be an upsetting time for family carers and intensify their feelings of grief, loss and guilt.

Ask for support during this transition – from friends, family or an Admiral Nurse. Perhaps consider reconnecting with hobbies, interests and family and friends you might have lost contact with while providing direct care for the person with dementia. Care homes can provide the opportunity to rebuild the spouse or parent/child relationship when the caring role is relinquished, and your primary family relationship can be re-established and strengthened.

Resuming previous relationships

Some things may improve for you when the person with dementia moves to a care home. It may be easier for you to relax and enjoy the visiting time spent with the person with dementia because you aren't having to undertake care tasks and you feel less tired. You may be able to simply 'be' with the person with dementia and resume a previous relationship for the first time in a long time.

Guilt when feeling unable to see the person with dementia

Some family members and friends may choose not to visit the person with dementia. It may be because they don't know what to say or do. Or they may be struggling to accept the change that has happened to their friend or relative. This may make you feel angry, but try to understand that this could be their way of grieving and you may not be able to change them. Remember also that they may be feeling guilt too because they feel like this. You could make suggestions such as visiting together, but try not to be angry. Keep them informed and tell them what you learned during your own visits.

Managing your feelings of guilt

A common statement I hear from family carers is 'I promised them I wouldn't put them in a home' or 'Mum and Dad want to remain in their own home'. There are inherent problems with these promises. Would the person with dementia ask you to make that promise if they knew in advance the sacrifices you'd have to make? I have seen family carers bend over backwards, quit their jobs, move house, add extensions and lose their marriages – all to keep these promises.

Hypothesise about what the person with dementia might have advised you if they could step out of their dementia and communicate with you. This might even include them offering their forgiveness of previously made promises to never place them in care.

Ask yourself these questions:

- What would you say to a close friend who was going through what you're going through?

- Would you want another family member to go through what you have to prevent *you* from going into a care home?

- Would you want *them* to feel guilty when they had tried their absolute best to keep their promises to you?

The likelihood is that the person would understand the complexities of what a family carer manages at home on a day-to-day basis. This might involve managing aggressive behaviours, surviving on only two hours of sleep a night, calling the police because the person with dementia has gone missing, dealing with multiple falls and hospital admissions, coordinating caregivers to come in and still feeling as though you're failing to look after them well enough. If someone else was experiencing this, you might say, 'I would have done the same thing.' It's exhausting just to think about, let alone do. Yet family carers often berate themselves, and tell themselves, 'I could/should have done more', when in reality they were barely hanging on.

- Acknowledge that guilt is a normal grief emotion, and while it is good to talk about it, don't let others minimise the validity of this emotion.

- Remind yourself that it is important for the wellbeing of the person with dementia that *your* life is fulfilling and meaningful outside of caring for them.

- Friendship, rest and self-care will do much to keep you going.

- Attend a local peer support group. Talking to others who are going through a similar experience to you can be helpful.

- Plan when you will visit, and when you do visit, take a meaningful item such as a photo album or plan an activity such as a walk, so you can spend quality time together.

- Remember that some days you may feel weighed down by guilt more than others. Be kind to yourself.

If, after doing the best you can, you feel immobilised by guilt, this could be a sign of depression and you should speak to your GP. Remember, there is a lot of support out there for you.

REFERENCES

Collateral Global (2021) 'CG Report 6: Effects of COVID-19 in care homes – a mixed methods review.' Accessed on 9/5/2022 at https://collateralglobal.org/article/effects-of-covid-19-in-care-homes.

Manthorpe, J., Samsi, K., Norrie, C. and Woolham, J. (2021) 'Caring in Covid-19: Personal assistants' changing relationships with their clients' family members.' *Journal of Long-Term Care*, 256–263. doi:10.31389/jltc.77.

Samsi, K., Cole, L. and Manthorpe, J. (2021) '"The time has come": Reflections on the "tipping point" in deciding on a care home move.' *Aging and Mental Health*. doi:10.1080/13607863.2021.1947963.

Vandrevala, T. and O'Dwyer, E. (2022) 'Perceptions and experiences of live-in carers: Why acknowledging versus neglecting personal identity matters for job satisfaction and wellbeing.' *Ageing and Society 42*, 1, 72–88. doi:10.1017/S0144686X20000744.

Wu, J., Mafham, M., Mamas, M.A., Rashid, M. *et al.* (2021) 'Place and underlying cause of death during the COVID-19 pandemic: Retrospective cohort study of 3.5 million deaths in England and Wales, 2014 to 2020.' *Mayo Clinic Proceedings 96*, 4, 952–963. doi:10.1016/j.mayocp.2021.02.007.

RESOURCES AND FURTHER READING

Reddall, C. (2021) *Anna and the Beast: The True Story of a Young Mum Diagnosed with Dementia, Aged 37*. Cheltenham: Goldcrest Books International.

Dementia UK
CHANGES IN CARE: CONSIDERING A CARE
HOME FOR A PERSON WITH DEMENTIA

www.dementiauk.org/get-support/diagnosis-and-specialist-suppport/
changes-in-care/choosing-a-care-home

Carers UK
The UK's only national membership charity for carers, Carers UK is both a support network and a movement for change.

www.carersuk.org

tide
together in dementia everyday (tide) offer a range of services and supports to carers of a person with dementia, such as support groups, training and campaigning.

www.tide.uk.net

Relatives & Residents Association
The national charity for older people needing care and the relatives and friends who help them cope.

www.relres.org

Rights for Residents

www.rightsforresidents.co.uk/resources

CHAPTER 16

'Do people living with dementia feel pain?'

PALLIATIVE CARE AND DEMENTIA

Nula Suchet

Palliative care, as it turns out, was a misnomer when it came to James's treatment. Whenever it was clear he was feeling pain, such as those times he was hoisted in and out of bed, I was told by the palliative care nurse that 'dementia patients don't feel pain'. This was followed by the assurance that after the procedure, 'he'll forget very quickly anyway'.

In the days that followed, James's condition fluctuated. On one day, he took a shower, smiled and ate his food, and I was almost fooled into thinking that he was on the mend. But I knew deep down that it wouldn't last. We had been living with James's dementia for 11 years now, and I knew he was ebbing away and losing his strength to fight.

I was in the supermarket, a trolley full of shopping, when I got a call from the care home: 'Come as soon as you can. James isn't going to make it.' When I arrived, James was shaking violently, and his carer told me that these fits were a sign his body was shutting down, unable to cope. Over time, he had received treatments that I felt were futile, such as course after course of antibiotics for his diarrhoea. I was filled with a fury that the antibiotics had all been pointless, and what he really needed was someone to kindly ease his discomfort. There were times when I begged the doctor to please ease his suffering. He told me James hadn't yet reached the *critical stage* and that we'd have to wait to let *it* happen naturally. One of the nurses tells me that Harold Shipman has a lot to answer for. Apparently, since his trial, rules around palliative care have been tightened, to the extent that some doctors no longer feel able to administer morphine in the kind of compassionate doses poor souls like James require.

Towards the end

I stayed with James for several days and nights. I could not eat or sleep and finally, when beaten, would return home each time and fall into bed but was unable to sleep. I would get up and call the care home every hour through the night to check on him. I was advised that I didn't need to call every hour as I needed to take care of myself and get some sleep. The night nurse assured me that if there was the slightest change, she'd call me. At 7 a.m. there's a call: 'I think you should come as soon as you can. James has deteriorated hugely in the last hour.' I watched James struggle to breathe. His ribcage looked as though it was going to break through the transparent skin of his chest. He plucked at the bedclothes in fear. The morphine patch prescribed by the doctor seemed woefully inadequate. How could I endure watching him suffer like this? James lingered on. I tried to be strong, but in the weeks that followed, James seemed to descend into a nightmare cycle of crisis after crisis. He had lost a lot of weight from chronic diarrhoea, and the four lots of drugs prescribed to treat it that did not work. He cried out each time the caregivers changed his incontinence pads but became so weak that even the effort to cry out was too much for him.

I was unprepared for how the final days would be. It got to the point where I demanded they call a doctor immediately. When he arrived, he admitted that James's deterioration was beyond what he'd expected, having seen him only four days previously. He said, 'It wasn't easy to gauge. James was difficult; he kept fighting back.' I questioned his belief that James was in any fit state to fight back. He conceded and immediately increased the morphine for the pain, and the midazolam to ease James's anxiety.

I didn't leave James's bedside for the next few weeks. In the final black hours of the final days, as death crept closer to him, I stroked his hair and told him how much I loved him and will never stop loving him. I longed to keep him beside me, but knew I must relinquish him to be free from this dreaded disease. He moved in and out of consciousness, and after days of constant vigilance and exhausted from lack of sleep, I was persuaded to go home and get some rest. I planned to go back in the morning. Dementia took James away in my absence. At 6.15 a.m. the telephone wakes me. 'It's the night nurse here, Nula. I'm sorry to tell you James has just passed away.'

The last months of James's life almost destroyed me. To this day, I'm haunted by James's horrendous last weeks and days of obvious pain and discomfort.

SPECIALIST COMMENTARY

Professor Elizabeth Sampson, Department of Psychological Medicine, Royal London Hospital, East London NHS Foundation Trust, and Division of Psychiatry, University College London

Nula's experiences are upsetting to read, and it is impossible to fully understand what she and James experienced during this time. Could these experiences have been different and how can we ensure others are not left with these memories? There were multiple points at which a palliative care approach could have better managed James's symptoms and supported Nula. This type of care is not necessarily complex or technical in nature, but it requires skill and sensitivity in its delivery. Nula is still haunted by her experiences, sadly reflecting the famous quote from Dame Cicely Saunders, the founder of the modern hospice movement:

How people die remains in the memory of those who live on.

What can palliative care offer for people dying with or from dementia?

It is important to appreciate what palliative care is (and is not). The World Health Organization (Davies and Higginson 2004, p.2) defines palliative care as:

an approach that improves the quality of life of patients and their families facing the problems associated with life-threatening illness, through the prevention and relief of suffering by means of early identification and impeccable assessment and treatment of pain and other problems, physical, psychosocial and spiritual.

Palliative care *does not* involve withdrawing care, giving less care or denying particular treatments, and can be applied for any condition that may limit a person's lifespan. There is widespread acceptance that it is highly relevant and often beneficial for people with dementia and their families. It emphasises a focus on assessing and managing distressing symptoms such as pain, while ceasing interventions that may not be in the long-term best interests of the person with dementia. So, for example, James may have not benefited from repeated courses of antibiotics for diarrhoea, and giving him these may have caused him distress and discomfort, whereas careful assessment and management of his pain and distress may have significantly improved his quality of life as he was dying. Palliative care takes a holistic approach, considering not just the physical but also a person's spiritual, psychological and social needs.

Improving pain management for people with dementia

A vital component of palliative care is to relieve suffering; pain management is an integral component of this. It is worrying that staff caring for James were of the belief that 'dementia patients don't feel pain'. There have been huge advances in our knowledge regarding pain and dementia over the last 20 years (Corbett *et al.* 2014). Numerous studies have found that people with dementia continue to feel pain but they may have difficulty in understanding what they are feeling, and in describing and locating the pain, and they may be unable to remember that they have been in pain and report this. The fact that their short-term memory for pain may lead them to forgetting this is no reason to ignore pain. A person with severe dementia lives in the moment, and if that is filled with pain, then there will be a profound impact on their quality of life. When the person is unable to understand or describe the pain they feel, they may still be aware of deeply distressing sensations that they are unable to express. This may lead, understandably, to resistance to being moved or hoisted, and then unfairly being labelled as uncooperative, agitated or even aggressive.

Clinicians may be concerned about the potential side effects of increasing the strength of analgesics in people with dementia.

However, studies have demonstrated that a stepwise approach to pain management – gradually moving from simple analgesics (such as regular paracetamol) to mild opioids (such as codeine) and then stronger opioids (e.g. morphine) – can be very effective in relieving distress and agitation caused by under-treated pain (Husebo *et al.* 2011). Similarly, feelings of breathlessness or distress secondary to constipation or delirium may all manifest as changes in the person's behaviour, and a palliative care approach, underpinned by careful assessment of symptoms, will identify and help to better manage these issues.

Palliative care and holding uncertainty
A recurrent theme from Nula's experiences is that of uncertainty. Accurately predicting how long someone with dementia is going to live is extremely difficult. There may be a gradual decline, interspersed by more sudden events such as falls or chest or urinary infections. Even during the last few days of life, the course of events can be unpredictable (Sampson *et al.* 2018). Palliative care offers an approach that holds and manages this uncertainty. Rather than focusing on how long someone may live, a palliative care approach assesses and attempts to address the person's needs across physical, spiritual, psychological and social domains. Clinicians who are skilled and confident in delivering palliative care can work with families and support them with this uncertainty. An honest and open way of addressing this could be: 'We may not be able to predict how long James may have left to live, but we will manage his symptoms and meet his needs as best as we can, so that in the remaining time he has left, we can relieve any distress and keep him comfortable.'

Discussing the end of life
Death remains a taboo in many societies. There are complex issues around discussing dying with dementia and end-of-life care. In the earlier stages of dementia, it is understandable that the focus should be on 'living well' with the disease. People with dementia and their families and friends will want to focus on the 'here and now'. The fact that dementia is a life-limiting illness is often not discussed around the point of diagnosis. Many people with dementia and their families do not wish to receive information about end-of-life care at this time.

However, as dementia progresses, it is difficult for professionals and families to find the 'right' time to discuss these important issues, and it is often left until there is a crisis or sudden deterioration – or, as happened with Nula and James, the discussion does not happen at all.

In summary

It is important to state that many people who die with dementia do receive good palliative care, and for some families, the experience of being with their relative who is dying with dementia can be peaceful and a chance to reflect on a life well lived. A step-change in care provision for people dying with dementia will require public support and engagement to drive policy changes, funding and how services are structured and delivered. Nula has bravely revisited a 'horrendous' period of her life to share her experiences and increase awareness of palliative care. Dementia is the most feared disease for people aged over 60 years, but there is less awareness of dementia as a life-limiting illness where a 'good death' is possible.

ADMIRAL NURSE ADVICE

Sharron Tolman, Consultant Admiral Nurse, Dementia UK

I am sorry to read of Nula's experience but thank her for sharing and highlighting this significant issue. It is so important we recognise dementia as a life-limiting illness. This can help people with dementia and their families to think ahead and consider the care they may want at the end of life, particularly when the person with dementia still has capacity to express their wishes. However, as we have heard from Professor Sampson, the trajectory of dementia can be unpredictable, so focusing on need(s), comfort and quality of life is key. Most of us do not want to think ahead too much, especially about when our life might end, and tend to live in the here and now. This can make it difficult to consider when it is the 'right' time to start to think about end-of-life preferences, but there are some key transition points and opportunities for advance care planning and end-of-life discussions (see Chapter 5) – for example, when people ask about death or dying, at a new diagnosis, when there are repeated hospital admissions, changes to care needs, multiple health conditions, deterioration in condition or signs of pain or distress. Advance care planning and considering goals of care can help the person with dementia and their family to feel more involved and prepared, in addition to supporting shared decision making and a good end-of-life experience. Expectant mothers and fathers routinely develop birth plans that may not always go to plan, but thinking and planning helps their understanding of the process and what to expect, as well as opening conversations and raising questions. So, thinking ahead is helpful and there are things you can do.

Comfort care

As outlined by Professor Sampson, management of a person's pain is central to palliative care, with the concept of 'total pain' embracing not just physical pain but also psychological, social and spiritual pain. As a person's dementia progresses into the advanced stages, pain may be expressed in different, non-verbal ways, such as through facial expressions, body movements, vocalisation (calling out or repeated noises) and changes in the person's interactions, behaviour and mood. Although self-reporting (where you directly ask the person if they are in pain) is the preferred or 'gold standard' for pain management, this is less likely to be effective when the dementia is in its more advanced stages and the person is nearing the end of their life. When asked if in pain, for example, a 'no' response may not be an accurate representation, so impeccable assessment is essential to ensure effective management of symptoms.

Creating a comfort care plan can help people, both care staff and family carers, involved in providing care for the person with dementia to understand how best to meet their physical, emotional, social and spiritual needs for comfort and help in managing any distressing symptoms. If the person with dementia is not able to express this themselves, a family carer may often be the person who knows them best, so their contribution to developing a comfort care plan is vital.

Consider what sort of environment makes the person feel comfortable, what makes them relaxed and happy, what brings emotional and physical comfort and what keeps them pain-free. This will be individual to everyone, and life story work can support this (see Chapter 1).

Doing this early in a person's experience of dementia is helpful to have in your 'toolbox' and to share with others involved in their care – for example, during a hospital admission where none of the hospital staff have knowledge of the person with dementia beyond what condition they are being admitted for. This may change over time, so it is helpful to see it as a plan you can adjust and tweak as long as it captures what matters. We often hold lifelong beliefs and values, which can still be strongly held even as dementia progresses. Examples may be if the person with dementia rarely visited a doctor or took analgesia, or used different words or behaviours to express their pain. This is valuable information that may help care staff to understand their responses to pain and distress and how best to manage this. These nuggets of information, capturing a person's individuality, values and beliefs including previous responses to pain or distress, are often only known to the person with dementia and/or close family and friends, so sharing this to develop end-of-life care plans is so important. Nula's story highlights the importance of this person-centred approach and the need to provide effective comfort care.

Building trust with families is crucial so that care staff can understand what matters most to family carers and the person affected by dementia – what may give them strength and comfort and what is required of care staff in supporting those needs. Opening communication is key, asking open questions to encourage expression of concerns. It is important for family carers to be able to relay to care staff what is important to them and how best they can be supported – for example, the person with dementia may have particular practices or routines they wish to follow. This could include prayer, reading or meditation or continuing to follow or practise an organised religion or faith. Understanding what, who or where they usually get their support from during difficult times may also help. This may be family, friends, occupation or hobbies and interests. Giving family carers several opportunities and invitations to share what else is on their mind may help to clarify concerns and worries and begin to formulate shared decision-making plans for care.

Nula's experience reminds us of the importance of us all having a shared understanding of what is happening to the person with dementia. Even in healthcare, we can often feel uncomfortable and avoid talking about death and dying, despite its inevitability, but this is not helpful when supporting families affected by dementia to understand what is happening. The unpredictable nature of dying with or from dementia may compound this with a concern for the professional carer that it may not be the 'right' time to talk about the person dying.

Some of the symptoms at end of life such as restlessness, confusion, hallucinations, sleeping more or not wanting to eat or drink may also be attributed to the dementia or progression of dementia, rather than the dying process itself, so openness to the possibility of dying and access to multi-professional support is vital to enable a good end-of-life experience and the valuable contribution of family carers.

Namaste Care

Namaste Care is a gentle, sensory approach which focuses on engaging with a person living with advanced dementia, where communication is often difficult. Communication using the Namaste Care approach is through the use of the senses – sound, touch, smell, taste and sight – to improve the quality of life of the person with dementia as they near the end of their life. Namaste Care can be incredibly helpful to family carers to maintain their sense of connection with the person with dementia, particularly when their verbal skills are reduced. Some examples may include:

- **Smell:** Use of familiar and favourite scents which stimulate positive memories can give a sense of relaxation, calm and wellbeing. This can include a scented room spray, a favourite perfume or aftershave, scented soap or hand cream, flowers, herbs and cooking smells such as bread, toast or other favourite foods which can then be combined with small tastes if this is possible.

- **Sound:** Favourite music from their teens, early 20s or significant events such as their wedding to evoke special memories. It could be a recording of a favourite musical instrument. Reading aloud can be very soothing – for example, from a book they may have particularly enjoyed in the past, poetry, rhymes or sharing a personal story from past holidays or special, memorable events.

- **Taste:** Small tastes of their favourite treats and drinks (if able to take by mouth). These could be related to the seasons (ice cream for the summer, treacle for bonfire night, etc.) or a theme (such as Christmas pudding and brandy butter). Baking and cooking use all the senses so enabling this where possible to enjoy tastes alongside smells and textures (such as baking bread) can give added pleasure.

- **Touch:** Hand, foot or scalp massages, applying face cream or make up, hand and feet washing, hair brushing and styling can be soothing and also provide a family carer a chance to engage with a person's sense of touch and of being touched. Simple hand holding or stroking a face or hand with soft fabrics can offer a similar sensory experience for the person with dementia. You can also place certain items into their hand and encourage manipulation by placing your own hands around them, using, for example, seasonal items such as acorns and conkers.

- **Sight:** Looking through old photographs or books with illustrations can evoke positive feelings. Where possible, spending time outside to enjoy nature, a garden, looking at the sky or seaside. If they are not able to go outside, bringing the outside in is an option – for example, using flowers and plants or items from the beach such as shells or sand. Other examples include wearing favourite clothes from different eras, exploring items from a past hobby, such as football memorabilia or looking at clips from favourite films, such as comedy sketches, musicals or nature.

As we have heard from Nula's experience, it is so important to understand an individual's life story and previous experiences to develop enjoyable sensory interactions, appropriate to the individual, which may reduce anxiety and distress for them. Families can often feel at a loss about how best to connect with someone with more advanced dementia and towards the end of life, but it is often the simple things that can have a significant impact on maintaining an emotional connection between you and the person with dementia. Similarly, these simple activities can give family carers a feeling of still being able to do something meaningful at a time when they can often feel helpless and that they have little control over the person's care.

REFERENCES

Corbett, A., Husebo, B.S., Achterberg, W.P., Aarsland, D. *et al.* (2014) 'The importance of pain management in older people with dementia.' *British Medical Bulletin 111*, 1, 139–148. doi:10.1093/bmb/ldu023.

Davies, E. and Higginson, I.J. (2004) *Better Palliative Care for Older People.* Copenhagen: World Health Organization Regional Office for Europe. Accessed on 9/5/2022 at https://apps.who.int/iris/handle/10665/107563.

Husebo, B.S., Ballard, C., Sandvik, R., Nilsen, O.B. and Aarsland, D. (2011) 'Efficacy of treating pain to reduce behavioural disturbances in residents of nursing homes with dementia: Cluster randomised clinical trial.' *BMJ 343*, d4065. doi:10.1136/bmj.d4065.

Sampson, E.L., Candy, B., Davis, S., Gola, A.B. *et al.* (2018) 'Living and dying with advanced dementia: A prospective cohort study of symptoms, service use and care at the end of life.' *PalliativeMedicine 32*, 3, 668–681. doi:10.1177/0269216317726443.

Suchet, N. (2019) *The Longest Farewell: James, Dementia and Me.* Bridgend: Seren Books.

RESOURCES AND FURTHER READING
Dementia UK
PAIN AND DEMENTIA

www.dementiauk.org/get-support/health-issues-and-advice/pain-in-dementia

UNDERSTANDING DYING

Dementia is a progressive condition, and everyone with the diagnosis will die with or from it. Understanding the changes that happen in the last days can help you feel more prepared for what to expect.

www.dementiauk.org/get-support/understanding-changes-in-dementia/understanding-dying

Namaste Care

Kendall, N. (2021) *A Namaste Care Activity Book.* London: Jessica Kingsley Publishers.

Kendall, N. (2020) *Namaste Care for People Living with Advanced Dementia: A Practical Guide for Carers and Professionals.* London: Jessica Kingsley Publishers.

Hospice UK
DEATH AND DYING: WHAT TO EXPECT

www.hospiceuk.org/information-and-support/death-and-dying-
what-expect

NOTE: Nula Suchet's piece is an edited version of an extract from her book *The Longest Farewell: James, Dementia and Me* (Seren, 2019).

Consultation Is Key

CONSULTATION

Professor Karen Harrison Dening

Key in developing the book was the consultation with families affected by dementia and recruiting any who wanted to contribute to the book sections. We explored several ways to recruit families, but given the experience, knowledge and networks of the editors, we ended up using a largely pragmatic approach. One of the editors (HH) was directly involved with two peer support groups in the Midlands. The first was Forget-Me-Nots,[1] which is a social group run by and for people with dementia, their partners and family carers, facilitated by Dementia UK and the University of Northampton, and the second was UnityDEM,[2] UnityDEM is a post-diagnostic support centre, another innovation of the University of Northampton, which aims to support families affected by dementia to build stronger social networks and to develop personal coping strategies. HH attended each of the two groups in person in February, before the social distancing measures of lockdown were enforced to contain the spread of the COVID-19 virus.

Another of the editors (KHD) was involved in establishing three peer support groups for people with dementia and family carers in Nottinghamshire facilitated by Trent Dementia,[3] a small charity in the East Midlands. Founded in Leicester in 2004, it began life as a member

1   www.northampton.ac.uk/research/research-centres/dementia-research-innovation-centre-ndric/northamptonshire-communities-of-practice/forget-me-nots-social-group
2   www.northampton.ac.uk/news/residents-benefit-from-unique-dementia-centre-that-helps-them-and-carers
3   www.trentdementia.org.uk

of a UK network of Dementia Services Development Centres and in 2014 moved to the Institute of Mental Health at the University of Nottingham. Each of the support groups was attended by KHD during the months of June and July 2020 where the concept of the book was presented and interest sought. The meetings were held virtually through an online platform as the COVID-19 pandemic was in full swing and all attendees observing social distancing.

A fourth source of consultation was through the activities of the third editor (CR) who has contributed to the book from a family carers' perspective. Her daughter, Anna, was diagnosed with behavioural variant frontotemporal dementia (BvFTD) in 2013 and died in 2017. She has written a book about this experience, and she is also a member of various groups working to promote palliative care for people with dementia. Over this time, she has developed a network of families similarly affected by BvFTD and has drawn on these contacts to support this book.

Lastly, we made two calls through the social media networks of Dementia UK to seek contributions from anyone who had some form of contact with the charity; this could be supporters of the charity, people with dementia and family carers, public with an interest in dementia, etc. The call was put out through Twitter, Facebook and LinkedIn on two separate occasions (March and July 2020).

We designed a format for the book chapters that followed the formula of starting with the issue or question as described by the family affected:

1. Each chapter would begin with a case study or issue that is or was experienced by the family, written either directly by the person with dementia and/or their family carer or, if preferred, 'ghost'-written by one of the book editors from their narrative. There was also the option to make their contribution but remain anonymous.

2. This would then be followed by a section that offered an 'expert commentary' to explain what may be happening, such as a neurologist if relating to changes in the brain, a psychiatrist or

psychologist for behaviours, a speech and language therapist for speech or swallowing problems, etc.

3. The last section would be from an Admiral Nurse and offer information, advice, tips and interventions that may help. This may also involve various other resources that the family may wish to consider. Finally, the Admiral Nurse will offer some key resources to support the issue.

While each of the groups and contacts received a verbal description of 'the ask', a brief survey tool was developed that people could take away with them to give the matter some thought. Following an introduction and a brief outline of the aim of the book and its proposed format (as detailed above), recipients of the survey were asked a few simple questions to guide the books' themes and to recruit possible contributors.

In helping us to plan this book could you consider the following questions:

1. Were there any problems or concerns that you had in the past that you would have liked help with or any that you would want help with now?

2. Did you receive or want an explanation of the reasons underlying any issues or behaviours you experienced? Would this have helped in your understanding or management of the behaviour/issue at the time?

3. We will be seeking people with dementia and/or their family to contribute to the case studies in the book; is this something you would be interested in doing?

Contact details of the editors were included so that anyone who was interested could make direct contact rather than wait for the next peer support group meeting. We received many responses from families who wanted to convey their stories, questions and issues. Of these, many were willing for us to use their story to form sections of the book.

THEMES

Although we did not undertake this work under the guise of formal research, we still wanted to ensure we gave full consideration to the rich narrative that respondents were giving us. Many of the issues and scenarios presented had several themes running through and many shared similar experiences. We have mapped the themes on to the trajectory of dementia from a point where there is a suspicion that all is not well, to diagnosis, and then throughout the many issues that arise when living with dementia. Many of the respondents did not want to contribute to the book by writing their own scenario, but in allowing us to support them to 'craft' their story, we tried to make sure that their experiences were sensitively and correctly reflected. We hope we have done these families justice through presenting the core themes to their stories.

Before the diagnosis

It is thought that people with dementia will usually present first to their general practitioner (NICE 2018) but many family carers who responded to our call found it difficult to persuade the person with the probable dementia to make a first appointment. Many families shared their experiences of what happened to them before the diagnosis – when it first started to feel that 'all was not well'. What was striking was that many described feeling alone during this period and spoke of the problems they encountered when trying to convince both the person's GP and other family members that 'something was not quite right' about your father, about my wife, about our brother. Some talked of disbelief when raising their concerns with other family members and of causing division. This stage was often marked as the first of the times the family carer started to feel their life was now a struggle and one in which they felt alone and/or isolated.

Getting the diagnosis

Diagnosing dementia requires taking a history of the person where this is suspected. The process of diagnosis involves evaluating for cognitive decline and impairment in daily activities of the person who is suspected of having dementia. This includes corroboration from a close friend or family member, in addition to a thorough mental status examination by a clinician to detect any impairments in memory, language, attention, visuospatial cognition such as spatial orientation, executive function and mood, as well as physical examination, laboratory testing and brain imaging (Arvanitakis, Shah and Bennett 2019; Sandilyan and Dening 2019). While the diagnostic process of dementia is not something that can be rushed as there is a lot to assess, measure and test to ensure accuracy, some felt their 'road to diagnosis' was a long one which, for some, extended into years. Several contributors had experience of young-onset dementia and spoke of going down many 'blind alleys' with instances of 'misdiagnosis' before eventually getting the diagnosis of dementia. Probably the most common differential diagnosis for a young-onset dementia is depression. Depression can masquerade as dementia and should always be considered; however, depression and dementia can coexist, and sometimes depression may precede dementia (Robinson, Tang and Taylor 2015). Although frequently misdiagnosed, Kuruppu and Matthews (2013) argue that a systematic approach in diagnosing young-onset dementia, as is the case for late-onset dementia, is reliant upon attainment of a detailed history, a collateral history from a family member or close friend, neuropsychological testing, laboratory studies and neuroimaging, which, if conducted well, may lead to an earlier and more accurate diagnosis. A small number of people delayed seeking help and therefore a delay in receiving the eventual diagnosis of dementia. In hindsight, they wished they had sought medical help sooner but at the time questioned what difference a diagnosis would have made. Clinical and care services argue that gaining the diagnosis as early as possible can help people with dementia gain earlier access to information, resources and support, make the most of their abilities and potentially benefit from drug and non-drug treatments available (SCIE 2015). The Social Care Institute for Excellence also proposes that an early diagnosis gives someone the chance to explain to family and friends the changes happening in their life. This would seem a reasonable outcome of an early diagnosis, but some of the contributors described the scenario where wider family members were mistrustful of the main carer's intention and refused to acknowledge or accept the changes in the individual.

Post-diagnostic support

Post-diagnostic support for people with dementia has been criticised for being insufficiently available, fractured and focused on managing crises rather than promoting wellbeing. Post-diagnostic support may encompass a range of supports that are offered to a person and their family once diagnosed with dementia (NICE 2018). The post-diagnostic support may be for a limited time or number of sessions following the diagnosis and continue for varying periods, sometimes until the death of the person with dementia. Providing support in the form of information, advice and access to services or social events is promoted as beneficial for people newly diagnosed with dementia and their families (Kelly and Innes 2016). However, what we heard was that post-diagnostic support was often difficult to access and failed to address an individual family's needs. Many spoke of having little or no information to guide them on what to expect – for example, behaviours that were highly predictable or just possible. Several would have preferred to be pre-warned about what they might experience, rather than learning after the event. Few families were informed about the possible life course of dementia, especially about what they may experience if the person lived into the advanced stages of the illness.

Interventions

It is difficult for families affected by dementia to understand the language used by health and social care professionals. Many reflected on a professional's use of the term 'intervention' when speaking of care of the person with dementia and failed to fully understand what this meant. Often, they were unaware that they (the person diagnosed with dementia and/or the family carer) were receiving an 'intervention' or, indeed, what potential 'interventions' were. Many interpreted 'intervention' to mean prescribed medications, with several giving detail of the distressing effects of such medications on the person with dementia. They stated that the medications prescribed 'turned out to be antipsychotics or benzodiazepines', and often these were used in times where there were extreme distress behaviours evident. Despite being recommended as first-line treatment (NICE 2018), non-pharmacological interventions are often under-prescribed (Cations *et al.* 2019), yet policy makers promote a reablement approach that promotes multi-disciplinary early intervention and ongoing access to non-pharmacological interventions such as occupational therapy, exercise and carer support. The response from the people we consulted was varied but, overall, they described a lack of confidence in caring, with an unfortunate lack of the 'intervention' of others and described their road in dementia care as a 'struggle set in the context of loneliness and a background of constant juggling'. The people we consulted largely framed their need for interventions and support in the context of the person they were caring for; several identified the feelings they were experiencing or had experienced, such as guilt, loneliness, social isolation and exhaustion, but many did not acknowledge or realise that their needs were very real and warranted a health and social care response. In Admiral Nursing, we often use an expression that aims to help family carers frame their own needs in parity with the needs of the person with dementia – 'the oxygen and the plane'. Parents (and carers of any kind) are advised to apply their own oxygen mask first to then be able to effectively support the person they care for to apply theirs. This analogy can often help a carer to consider that they have tangible needs and that it is OK in some instances to put their own needs before those of the person they care for.

When problems occur

As we have already heard, many spoke of a response to their needs only when they had 'hit the wall of a crisis', and the crises reflected upon were manifold. They detailed relating to some of the physical health problems they experienced, where the person with dementia had another co-existing condition or where they developed an infection that 'upset the apple cart'. Often mentioned were how they had to manage delirium as a result of a urinary tract infection or how to help a person up after a fall and 'have the confidence to assess for any injuries themselves so as not to bother the ambulance service again'. As clinicians, we know that older adults with dementia, even early-stage dementia, have an increased risk of falling, with risks to their health and quality of life (Lach, Harrison and Phongphanngam 2016). There are interventions and activities available with some potential to reduce falls, but how is this knowledge transferred to families affected by dementia? Similarly, as clinicians, we understand the identification and management of delirium superimposed on dementia. It is an acute medical illness that is difficult to diagnose because of the similarities of the symptoms to dementia, yet it can hugely contribute to the distress of the person with dementia as well as the family carer (Parrish 2019). But what does this all mean for families? How can we better translate the many and varied potential for problems to occur into a language that is acceptable and in a format that is bite-sized and accessible? The mantra that is used in dementia care education and practice is that 'when you have seen one person with dementia, you have seen one person with dementia'. Despite commonalities in factors, signs and symptoms, all are individuals and experience their dementia in their own inimitable way.

Legal issues

One final but significant theme that emerged was information and guidance on a range of legal issues. There were several scenarios offered that portrayed where good legal advice and information were provided but came too late to act upon as the person with dementia had already lost the mental capacity to be active in the process. This was of particular note when discussing their wishes and preferences for healthcare at the end of life, with some family carers feeling the 'burden of decision making'. Dementia is a life-limiting condition, so it is essential that soon after the diagnosis, families are given timely information about the course of dementia and the care options (Sampson and Harrison Dening 2020). They need to understand that a palliative approach to care might be appropriate and does not mean abandonment of the patient. They might also want clarification about their role in the decision-making process, especially if withholding or withdrawing life-prolonging measures are considered.

IN SUMMARY

It is essential to tailor care, support and interventions to the needs of families affected by dementia to ensure they are both targeted and relevant. This should be no different when preparing a guide such as this. We have taken time to discover the issues of relevance to people with dementia and their families and tailored our responses accordingly, seeking the narratives and stories of families affected by dementia to guide each section, a specialist in each of the fields that arise and then matching a skilled Admiral Nurse to offer advice and support.

We are very grateful to all of the many people who have contributed to this book. It can be a difficult task to bring together and edit each contribution to deliver 'the whole' while retaining individual styles and practice; however, we feel each still makes its own unique contribution.

REFERENCES

Arvanitakis, Z., Shah, R.C. and Bennett, D.A. (2019) 'Diagnosis and management of dementia: Review.' *JAMA 322*, 16, 1589–1599. doi:10.1001/jama.2019.4782.

Cations, C., Radisic, G., de la Perrelle, L., Laver, K.E. and The Agents of Change Collaborative Group (2019) 'Post-diagnostic allied health interventions for people with dementia in Australia: A spotlight on current practice.' *BMC Research Notes 12*, 559. doi:10.1186/s13104-019-4588-2.

Kelly, F. and Innes, A. (2016) 'Facilitating independence: The benefits of a post-diagnostic support project for people with dementia.' *Dementia 15*, 2, 162–180. doi:10.1177/1471301214520780.

Kuruppu, D.K. and Matthews, B.R. (2013) 'Young onset dementia.' *Seminars in Neurology 33*, 4, 365–385. doi:10.1055/s-0033-1359320.

Lach, H.W., Harrison, B.E. and Phongphanngam, S. (2016) 'Falls and fall prevention in older adults with early-stage dementia: An integrative review.' *Research in Gerosssntological Nursing 10*, 3, 139–148. doi:10.3928/19404921-20160908-01.

National Institute for Health and Care Excellence (NICE) (2018) 'Dementia: assessment, management and support for people living with dementia and their carers.' NICE guideline [NG97]. Accessed on 9/5/2022 at www.nice.org.uk/guidance/ng97.

Parrish, E. (2019) 'Delirium superimposed on dementia: Challenges and opportunities.' *The Nursing Clinics of North America 54*, 4, 541–550. doi:10.1016/j.cnur.2019.07.004.

Robinson, A.L., Tang, E. and Taylor, J.-P. (2015) 'Dementia: Timely diagnosis and early intervention.' *BMJ 350*, h3029. doi:10.1136/bmj.h3029.

Sampson, E.L. and Harrison Dening, K. (2020) 'Chapter 27: Palliative and End-of-Life Care.' In T. Dening, A. Thomas, R. Stewart and J.-P. Taylor (eds) *Oxford Textbook of Old Age Psychiatry*. Oxford: Oxford University Press.

Sandilyan, M.B. and Dening, T. (2019) 'Diagnosis of Dementia.' In K. Harrison Dening (ed.) *Evidence-Based Practice in Dementia for Nurses and Nursing Students*. London: Jessica Kingsley Publishers.

Social Care Institute for Excellence (SCIE) (2015) 'Why early diagnosis of dementia is important.' Accessed on 9/5/2022 at www.scie.org.uk/dementia/symptoms/diagnosis/early-diagnosis.asp.

Index